How to Start a
Makeup Artist
Business from Home

Published by Saffron Publishing Ltd

http://saffronpublishing.com

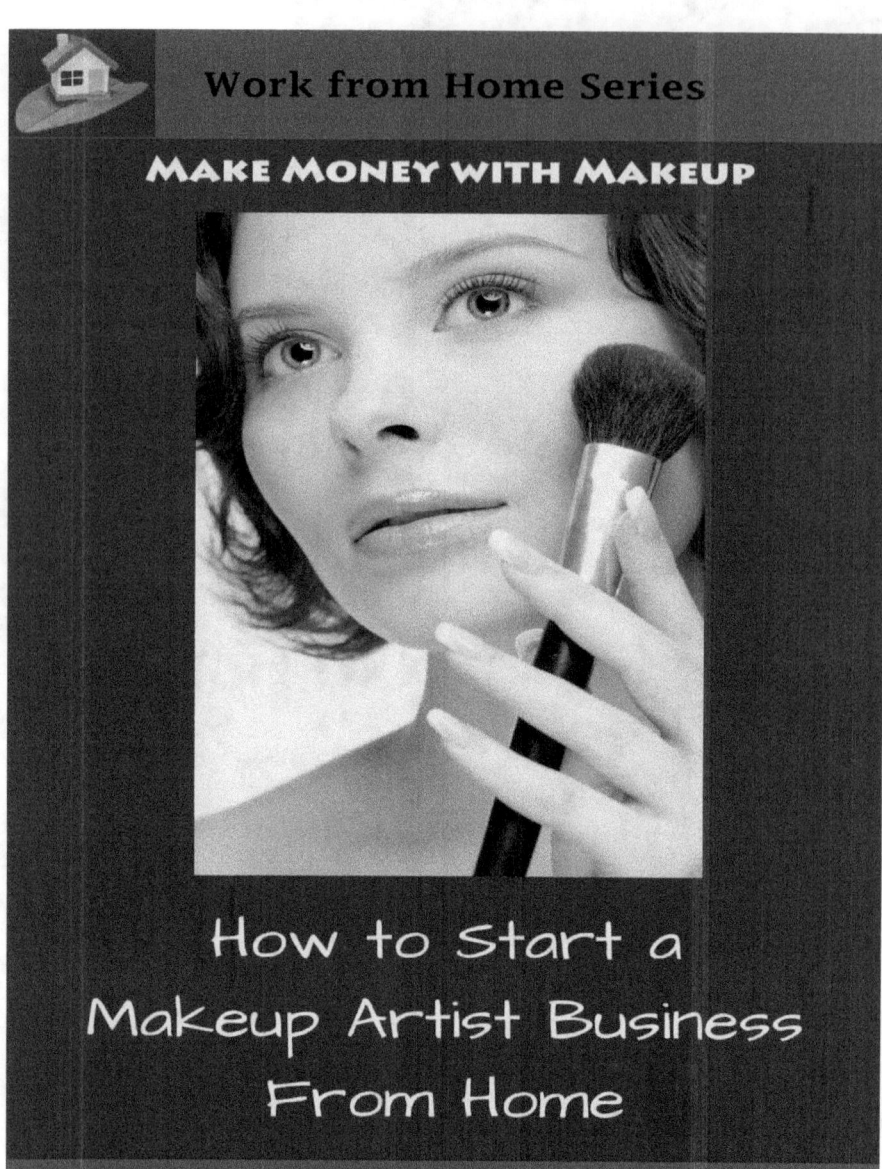

Work from Home Series

MAKE MONEY WITH MAKEUP

How to Start a Makeup Artist Business From Home

Anne Perez

Get Your FREE Gift …See Page 154

Get Your FREE Gift ...See Page 154

Dedication

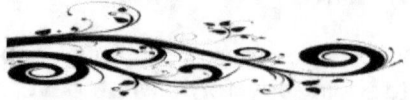

To all of you passionate about makeup and wanting to follow your dreams to become a makeup artist

Content

Get Your FREE Gift …See Page 154

Get Your FREE Gift ...See Page 154

Get Your FREE Gift ...See Page 154

Introduction

I wrote this book for those of you who would love to make money making others look and feel good about themselves but don't believe that it's possible! I am proof that it is.

As a child I was such a 'tom boy'. I would love to play football with the boys, climb trees, and get into mischief. Look pretty? Why? That was my twin sister! She loved makeup and pretty dresses and fashionable shoes and despaired at my lack of concern for such things.

If people who knew me as a child had known that I would be the one who became a makeup artist they would have laughed and said no way! I would have laughed too! However, circumstances conspired and I spent 20 years in the cosmetics field both as a makeup artist and building large teams for 2 cosmetic giants. I now spend my time helping others build successful businesses. I hope to help you too.

A career in Makeup Artistry is a chance to showcase your creativity. You will get paid to help people look fabulous and feel great about how they look. It's very rewarding,

Get Your FREE Gift ...See Page 154

the hours are flexible, the job is fun and top makeup artists earn a great deal of money for their services.

No matter who you work with your job is to help people look gorgeous. You touch lives with glamour and beauty. The smile on people's faces says it all. When they look good they feel good and their confidence becomes such that they feel they can do anything they set their minds to.

If you're looking for a fun, exciting, glamorous new career why not start a Makeup Artist Business. You can use your creative flair to help women look and feel beautiful. It will make you feel good too when you see their excitement at the look you just created for them.

I assume since you bought this book that you already have the desire to set up your own business making others look beautiful. I'm not going to spend time covering things that you already know.

You know WHY you're here, so let's just get to that purpose. Sound good?

So, what I'd like to do in the beginning of this book is to give you some foundational principles that we are going to build upon as we get into the practical aspects of setting up your own makeup artist business.

Get Your FREE Gift ...See Page 154

So, the first thing we are going to look at are some of the ingredients that I believe are necessary in order to build a successful makeup artist business of your own.

Ingredients for Success as a Makeup Artist Business Owner

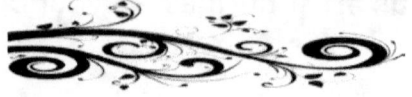

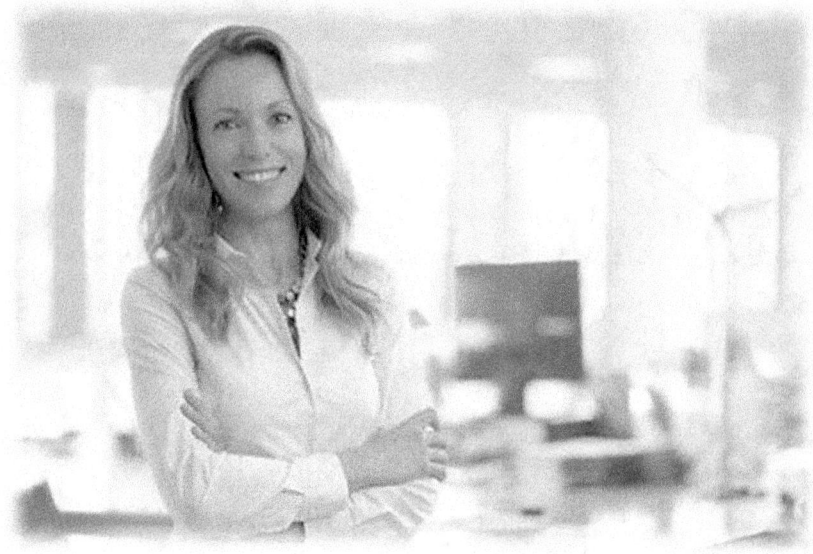

Having your own makeup artist business is very exciting, although at the beginning a little daunting when you are getting everything set up. I always feel that some understanding of what it will take to become successful really helps when starting out. Being a makeup artist and owning your own successful makeup artist business offers great rewards but you must be prepared and committed to the role. Determining if you ready to start your own makeup artist business at the beginning of your journey is time well spent.

The first thing to do when you start out is to evaluate your strengths and weaknesses as a potential owner and manager of a small business.

Are you a self-starter?

As the owner of a business you make the decisions. You don't take orders from anyone else and you decide how, when and what your business will look like and what you will offer your clients. It will be entirely up to you to decide on what type of makeup artistry you want to do, how many hours you're prepared to work, whether to employ others in the business or not. You will also find the clients and offer them services, which you yourself decide upon. You make the decisions. I, myself love the freedom of making my own decisions, setting my own hours and working where and with whom I choose. Is that something you want to do?

Business ownership can be exciting, but it's also a lot of work. In the early days especially there is a lot to do to get your business up and running and attracting clients. Are you up for the challenge?

Do you get along well with other people?

When you run your own makeup artist business you will meet and need to develop working relationships with many different types of people including customers, sales people, staff, bankers, lawyers, accountants, or consultants. There will be times when you may have to deal with a demanding client, an unreliable vendor, or a cranky receptionist if your business needs them. How well do you think you would cope in these situations?

Do you plan and organize well?

Research shows that poor planning is responsible for most business failures. Good organization of finances, inventory, schedules, and customer records can help you avoid many pitfalls. We will be looking more into these aspects of running a business later in the book.

Is your ambition strong enough?

Running a makeup artist business can wear you down emotionally. Some business owners burn out quickly from having to carry all the responsibility for the success of their business on their own shoulders. Strong motivation will help you survive slowdowns and periods of burnout.

The first few years of a new business can be hard on family life. It's important for family members to know what to expect and for you to be able to trust that they will support you during this time. There may also be financial difficulties until the business become profitable, which could take a while.

I find that being aware of problems that may arise makes it easier to handle them when they come along. If you truly want to run your own makeup artistry business you can do it. Just keep going despite the obstacles that may get in your way.

There's nothing more rewarding than being in charge of your own life: deciding when and where to work and when to take breaks and holidays, not having to ask

Key Personality Skills of the Successful Makeup Artist

1. **Confidence**
2. **A Friendly Attitude**
3. **The Desire to Help Others**
4. **Great Customer Service**
5. **Well Groomed**
6. **The Ability to Keep Calm**
7. **Patience**
8. **Creative**
9. **Communication Skills**

permission and deciding on who you work with. However you are also in charge of your income: finding new clients, keeping them happy and growing your business.

Get Your FREE Gift ...See Page 154

Now you're sure that you want to start your own makeup artistry business let's look at the key personality skills of the successful makeup artist. Skills that if developed will ensure your business stands out from your competition

Confidence

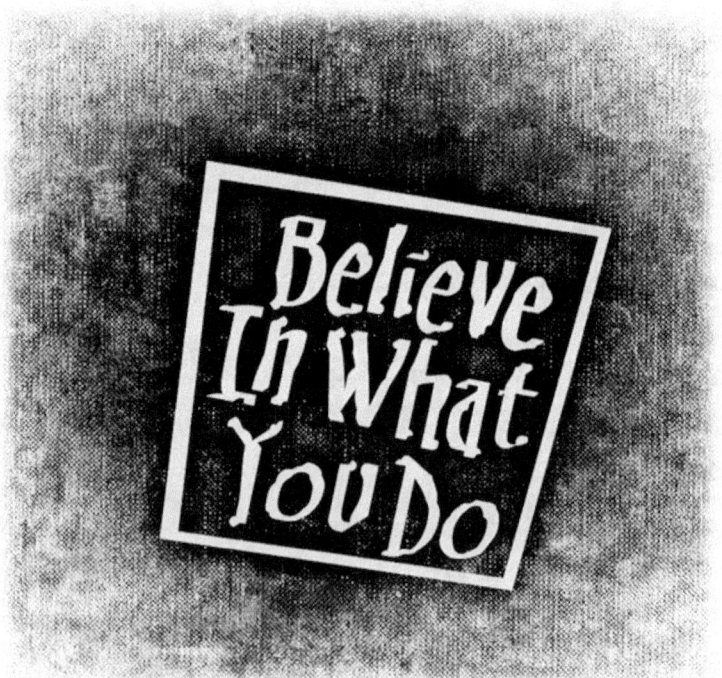

When you apply makeup you need to assure your client that you are skilled at what you do. Makeup application is very personal and intimate. You are often meeting people for the first time when you apply their makeup. They do not know you so you have to build up trust with them very quickly.

Being confident in what you do goes a long way to helping your client relax and let you do your work. If they sense that you are nervous and unsure about what you are doing they will get nervous too. Not a good combination for a good result.

Approach your clients calmly, reassuringly and confidently. Let your clients feel that they are in capable hands and they are more likely to relax and enjoy having their makeup done.

A Friendly Attitude

A makeup artist has to be a 'people person'. If you don't enjoy being around people then it's probably not a good career choice for you. People can sense if you're friendly, sincere and honest and are more likely to hire you if you are pleasant to be around.

A friendly and cheerful attitude around your clients will also encourage future business as your clients will refer you to others and ask you back themselves. Word of mouth is the cheapest and easiest way to grow your business.

The Desire to Help Others

As a makeup artist you're working to make other people look great and feel good about themselves. You're not usually in the limelight but you'll get great reward from making others feel happy, confident and excited.

Great Customer Service

Applying makeup is very intimate and you need to make the client feel at ease immediately. They need to trust you and believe that you'll do a great job. You need to be relaxed, friendly, warm and reassuring. It's critical that you build good customer relationships. Be accessible and approachable.

Well Groomed

You'll work very close to the client so you need to have a clean, well groomed appearance. It's important to wash daily, and use deodorants. Use cologne and fragrances sparingly. It's important not to smell of smoke too – so beware if you smoke

Artistic talent

The most successful makeup artists are artists first and consider the face their canvas and makeup their paints. It helps to understand and appreciate colour Have an objective eye and be visual in nature.

The Ability to Keep Calm

Have you heard the saying "keep calm and carry on"? Well that certainly applies in the case of being a makeup artist.

You are often racing against the clock to get the work done. You'll sometimes feel that you're in an impossible situation. Too much to do, too little time, interruptions, stressed models or brides: a hectic environment. Be prepared for all of them! It's so important to keep your cool.

Staying calm under the pressure will help other people around you and enable you to do a great job despite what's going on in your environment.

Flexible about the work

A Makeup Artist often works on different assignments on a daily basis so needs to very flexible. One day you might be working with a bride and her wedding party and the next making up models for a fashion show.

Patience

There may be times when you're waiting around in between clients. You may also have been hired for the day to create a look and then to do touch-ups when required. Patience is an essential skill at such times.

Be patient also in your attention to detail: In television and film, a challenge is often posed by scenes being shot out of sequence. The Makeup Artist needs to make sure that the actor's makeup looks the same in all shots. Photos and detailed notes can help jog your memory.

Get Your FREE Gift ...See Page 154

A Steady Hand helps too: To apply makeup consistently and evenly and to duplicate a specific look from one eye to the other a steady hand is a great asset.

Creative

As a Makeup Artist you're an Artist not a technician. You notice when makeup is put on poorly. You have good hand eye coordination. You're used to experimenting with colour and different makeup to see what you can create.

Good Communication Skills

It's really important that you can communicate with your client. The client needs to be able to understand you and also to know that you are listening to what they want.

Makeup artists need to be able to express themselves well. To tell clients what they can do and how they will do it in a professional manner. First impressions are really important and effective communication is essential right from the beginning in order to get the job.

Think about how you talk to other people both in person and on the phone! Ask other people how you

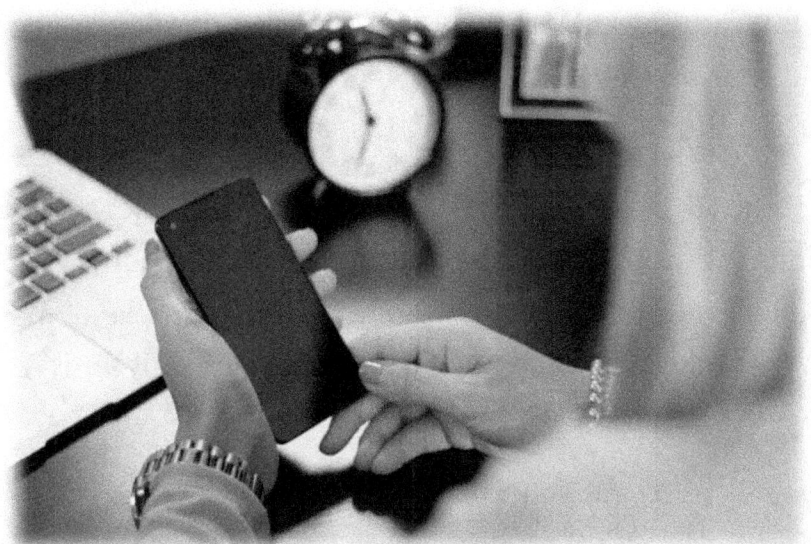

sound and about the words you use. If that's not possible try recording yourself! Would you hire you?

Do you listen to what your client is saying? In order to have a successful outcome the client must feel that you are listening to what they want. You may have a vision as to what you think would look best but does your client have other ideas?

As the professional you know more than your client but it's important to use your skills as a makeup artist to interpret your client's wishes in the way that will make them look the best possible.

If you're not sure what your client is asking summarize what you believe they are saying which will ensure both you and the client are thinking the same way.

It's a good idea as a makeup artist to become a good reader of body language and facial expressions. In a private rather than a commercial setting the client may not tell you that you've done a good job but wait until you leave to wash the makeup off.

If you give complimentary consultations it's especially key to recognize whether the client is truly happy with the result or not. You don't want to lose the business. It just might be that the client is uncomfortable asking you to change anything. In a more commercial setting you will be told that the makeup is not right.

As well as being in tune to the body language and facial expressions of your client it's a good idea to understand what signals you are giving off too. You want to project confidence and competence in how you do your work. If you're not sure ask a friend to watch you and provide feedback.

These skills of the successful makeup artist that we've been discussing can be developed by practice and by developing your technical skills. The more capable you are in your makeup artistry technique the more confident you will be.

"Be a very personable individual, and caring, because...we're in a very caring business"

Marvin Westmore

Do you have the qualifications that you need?

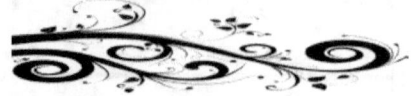

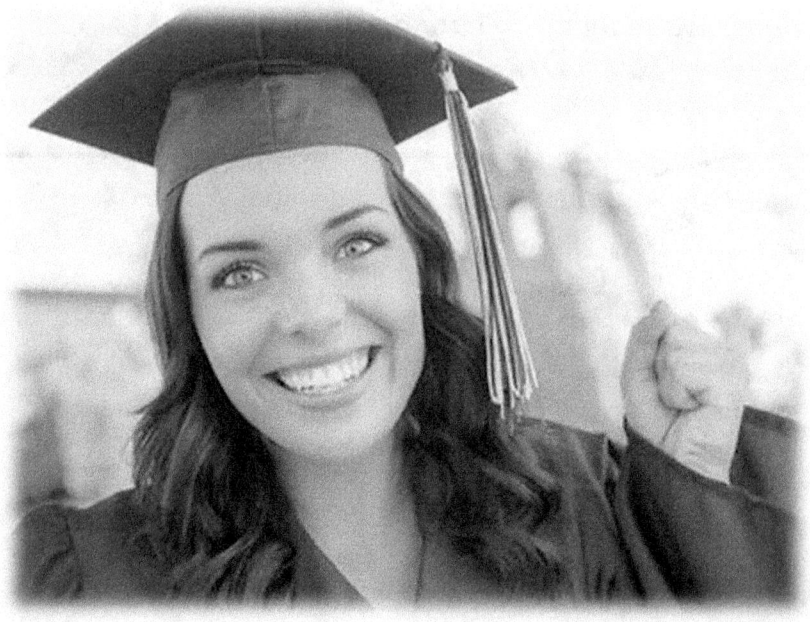

It's important during the beginning stages of setting up a makeup artist business to research what qualifications and licenses you need.

Find out if you need to get a cosmetologist licence to apply makeup professionally in your area. Where this is not a requirement it will be a lot faster to start a makeup artist business.

At the time of writing a makeup licence is not required in the UK but a licence requirement varies state to state in the USA. Be safe and research online to find out the requirement where you live. A simple search on Google should provide you with the answer.

Where a cosmetology licence is required you'll need to attend an accredited course. Look into local makeup artistry courses that suit you and that are accepted by the licensing board in your area. There are different rules and regulations depending on where you live.

Where a cosmetology license is not required it is still advisable to learn or update your makeup application skills. You can attend college courses, take online courses or teach yourself by using the multiple resources to be found online.

In addition you could join a direct sales company to increase your skills. Mary Kay Cosmetics for example holds many training sessions in product knowledge and cosmetics application.

Whilst getting your qualifications, where you need them, you can still start building up your business so when you graduate you can launch your business immediately.

In the meantime you can earn extra income by teaching makeup application skills or selling a cosmetics product line such as Avon or Mary Kay Cosmetics. Doing so will provide you with product knowledge and even build a client list to offer your services to once qualified.

You can earn while you learn and in addition you have a product range you can sell to your clients. On many occasions in my makeup artistry business I was asked by clients what products I used and they were extremely happy when I was able to provide them with the products.

Should I go to Beauty School?

I often get asked whether to be a makeup artist you have to go to beauty school. I myself never formerly studied makeup nor did many of the working makeup artists that I know. Many top makeup artists are self-taught and just enjoyed and discovered a talent at applying makeup, others went to makeup or cosmetology school. Either way a passion for colour, art and people is a prerequisite.

If you're interested in learning in a formal, structured setting then a makeup course, programme or school may be the right thing for you to do. Almost every area of the country will have a cosmetology programme that offers a makeup course. You may even find other established makeup artists in your area that offer seminars or workshops for aspiring artists. Since formal schooling is a big expense up front be sure to ask about what type of makeup techniques the programme will cover, the credentials of the instructor and the tools and supplies that will be provided e.g., if you're interested in learning bridal makeup techniques and the course is geared toward another type of makeup you'll want to know before you sign up. Some courses may require that you have a full makeup kit, others may provide you with some makeup and tools so ask what products and tools are needed beforehand. Ask questions before you enroll on the course!

Enrolling in a makeup class or programme is also an opportunity to network with others and make connections with other makeup artists which in turn may lead to work.

Learning on your own:

There are lots of video tutorials, beauty blogs, books and magazines showing lots of ways to apply makeup successfully. It is important to practice on friends and families and ask for honest feedback from every person you touch.

For more information on studying to become a makeup artist take a look at the resource section at the back of the book and visit our resource page at http://makemoneywithmakeup.com

Makeup may not change the world or even your life, but it can be a first step in learning things about yourself you may never have discovered otherwise.   *Kevyn Aucoin*

Planning Your Business

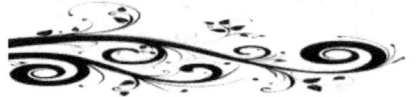

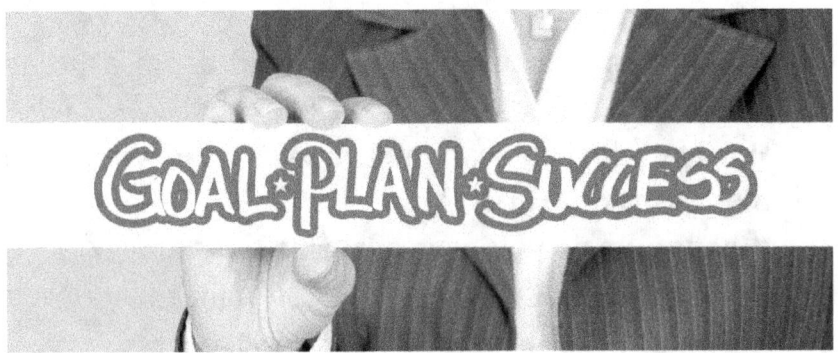

I know! I know! A business plan! Yuck! I just want to do makeup? Unfortunately without planning your makeup business is more likely to fail. If you want to succeed in business you need to plan your steps. It doesn't have to be difficult though and you can create a plan in just a couple of hours! Spend the time now and you'll reap the rewards later!

A business plan is simply a description of your business and how you plan to start and operate your business. It involves:

- A description of your business
- Your financial plan for your business

- How you're going to find customers
- How you're going to run the business.

Questions to ask yourself include:

- Do you want to go mobile or work from a home studio?
- How far do you want to travel if you work as a mobile makeup artist?
- What hours do you have available?
- How many hours per week do you want to work?
- How many clients do you want each year?
- How much money do you have to invest in your business?
- Where do you see your business in 6 months, 1 year, and 5 years?
- What kind of clients do you want
- What services will you offer and at what prices
- Will you be offering products in addition to services in your business?
- What is the legal structure of your business?
- How will your business be different from others already out there in the area?

The idea of creating a business plan may seem daunting but I've included a template on the accompanying website at http://makemoneywithmakeup.com that you can download and follow to easily put one together.

The first part of your business plan is all about your business and about you. Let's get started...

If the business is you then put your name down as the business owner and the business name. Next write down what you would love to accomplish in your business. Is there an area of makeup you would like to specialize in for example bridal makeup? How big do you want your business to get? How many clients would you ideally love to have? How busy do you want to be? Do you want to work just a few hours a week or take as much work as possible? Be as specific as you can since the answer to these questions will help you when it comes to finding the customers you want!

About Yourself

The second page is about you. Why do you want to be a beauty professional? Why do you want to have your own business? It's really important to know why since it's your why that will keep you going when times are difficult. When you're tired or things aren't working out as planned! As with everything you'll have good days and bad days even when you're doing what you love!! Knowing your why will stop you from quitting too soon.

Products and Services

The third page of this section is about your products and services. What services will you be offering clients? Will you be offering any products as well? Which brand? Where will you get your supplies?

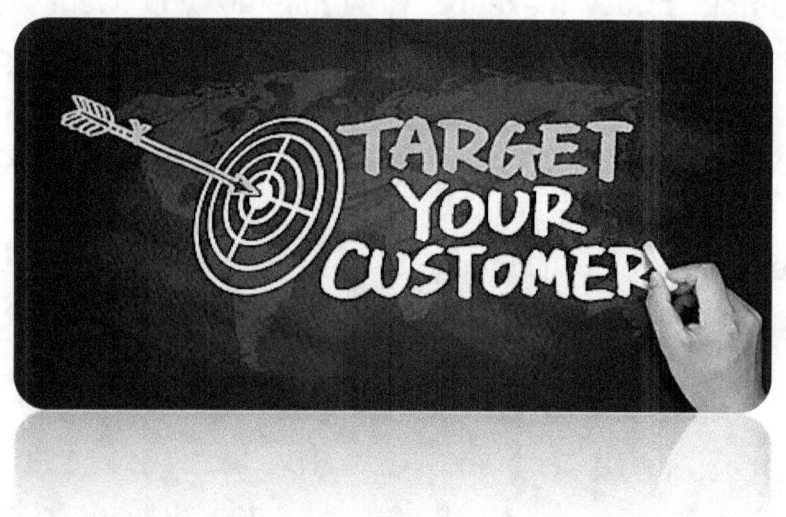

Finding Customers

In this section of the business plan we look at who is your typical customer or if you're just starting out who is your ideal customer? It's not everyone! I've heard it said by many small business owners that their market is 'everyone'. They are afraid that if they limit their pool of potential customers then their business will suffer. In reality the opposite is true. Choosing to specialize in offering products or services to a certain type of customer will result in more success for your business. Why is this: Simply because it is much easier to determine where and how to promote your business. You'll spend less time and money and have more success by selecting your customers from a certain sub sector of the population. Do you want to specialize in fashion makeup, bridal makeup, corrective makeup or glamour makeup for instance?

Specializing in a certain type of customer will also help you identify their needs better and you will sell more of your products and services to them because you are providing what they are looking for.

Researching the Competition

Continuing on the theme of marketing this section of the business plan is all about your plans for promoting your business. We'll be looking at marketing in more detail later in the book but for now just jot down your current ideas on how you are going to spread the word about your makeup artistry business.

Next is a section all about your competitors. It's a good idea to see who else is offering similar products and services to you and how they are finding customers. Knowing about your competition will help you decide how to set up your own offerings to customers. What are they doing well: what can you do that is similar? What are they doing poorly: How can you do it better? What is missing that people are asking for? Can you offer that product or service in your business?

What is so good about your Products and Services?

What makes you different from all the other beauty businesses in your town? What do you offer your clients that is different from your competitors? I don't mean just your products or services but how you make your clients feel. There may be a lot of people with similar technical skills to you but what can you do or what is it about you that encourages clients to buy from you and potential customers to come to you?

Do you have a bubbly personality? Are you warm and friendly? Do you offer exceptional customer service? Are you reliable? How do you benefit your clients? Why do they like you?

Think about yourself for a minute! What kind of service would you enjoy receiving if you were the client? What personal qualities in the makeup artist would be important to you? These could provide your own uniqueness. Your own USP (unique selling proposition) Again, we are only touching on this here but we'll look in more detail at branding and creating your own USP later in the book.

How Are You Going to Run Your Business?

Simply stated the logistics is how you are going to run your business. How will you offer your services as a makeup artist? Who are your suppliers? What equipment, tools and products do you need to run your business? How will you get paid? What insurance and legal requirements are there?

Costs and Pricing Strategy

The final section of your business plan is pricing. How to price your products and services can be a difficult decision to make and it has a lot to do with how you want to be seen in the market place. Do you want to offer premium, quality services? If so, then price yourself at the higher end and look for clients who have money to spend and are basing their decision on quality not price.

Alternatively charge lower prices and provide a budget service. However, make sure you are covering the costs of your supplies, tools, products, travel, professional development e.g. education and your time. Time is a resource in short supply so take it into consideration when pricing your services.

I suggest when pricing your services that you research the rates of your competitors and then place your own rates within the upper 10% of your competitors' price range.

In addition, create packages. Packages create a higher perceived value in the eyes of your clients. Don't charge 'by the hour' but by different packages, adding services to each package as the price goes up. For example you could offer a bridal package to a future bride which has a range of options to choose from a simple makeup look to the full works.

In addition to creating a business plan it's a good idea to think about how and where to set up a home office.

Setting up a Home Office

You'll need to find a place where you can handle the administrative side of your business such as Making phone calls, following up on emails, keeping records and storing supplies.

Ideally you'll have a place where you can work undisturbed even if it's in the corner of a room that you can put screens around.

Useful equipment includes a computer, laptop or tablet for record keeping, accounts, marketing, keeping in touch with customers and more. A fast internet connection is helpful since it enables you to get your work done more quickly in the office. An all in one printer is a useful item to make copies of contracts, marketing materials and invoices and for scanning items. In addition you might want to consider getting a second phone to separate your business from your personal life. As your business grows this becomes more important.

If you want to succeed in business you need to plan your steps. It doesn't take long to do but it's really worth doing if you want to build a successful makeup artistry business.

Get Your FREE Gift ...See Page 154

For more information on planning your makeup artist business take a look at the resource section at the back of the book and visit our resource page at http://www.makemoneywithmakeup.com

Taking Care of Bits and Bobs: Legal, Insurance, Money, Tax

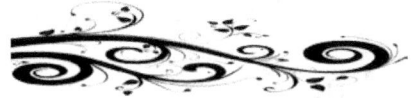

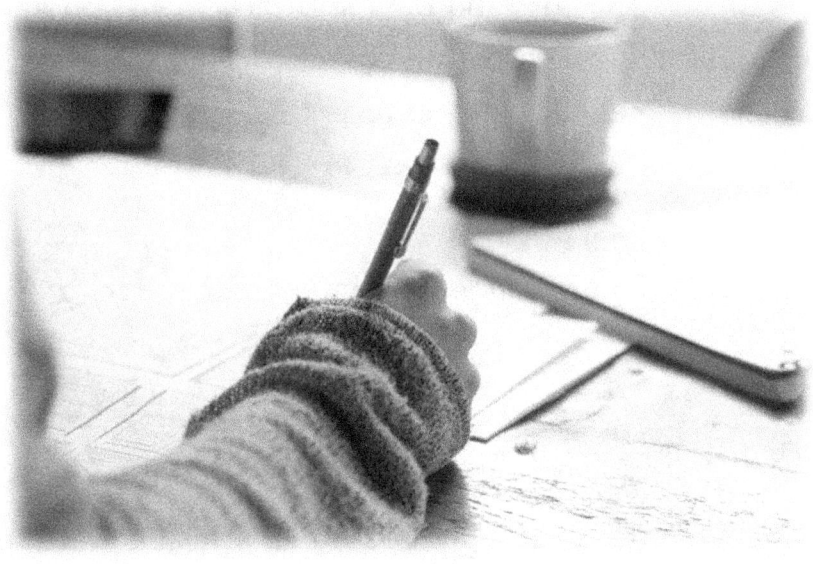

I must stress right at the beginning of this chapter that I am not a professional lawyer, insurance agent, tax agent or accountant. This book is for informational purposes only and is based on my experience running a makeup artistry business. If advice concerning legal or related matters is needed, the services of a fully qualified professional should be sought. This book is not intended for use as a source of legal or accounting advice. You should be aware of any laws which govern business

Get Your FREE Gift ...See Page 154

transactions or other business practices in your country and state.

Decide on a Name

To be unique and to stand out from the crowd you and your business need to be memorable. Spend some time choosing a name that is memorable. One that is:

- Easy to remember
- Easy to spell
- Web Friendly (an important consideration these days)

Check that the name:

a) Can be registered as a domain name (available website name)

b) is available on social media sites

Tip: Do you want to be known in a specific geographic area? Include that area in your name (this will help in being found more easily online)

Legal

If you haven't done so already research what qualifications and licences you need to work on clients. Do you need a cosmetology licence to apply makeup professionally in your area? At the time of writing a licence is not required in the UK to be a makeup artist but a cosmetology licence requirement varies state to state in the USA. If you sell your beauty products you may need a resale license.

Research what legal requirements need to be fulfilled to set up your business where you live. What are your tax obligations? Who do you need to contact in regards to becoming self-employed or running your own business?

In the USA you'll need a federal tax ID number. Some cities may require you to obtain a business license or local tax number so be sure to do your homework for that area. Most states require any type of business to obtain a license to legally operate within the state. Many makeup artists are considered independent contractors or self-employed business owners. Speak with a representative at your state or town business office to determine what type of business license you may need for your makeup business. You may find the following link helpful http://www.simplefilings.gov-tax.com/

In the UK you need to inform HMRC that you are self-employed. You also need to consider National Insurance and VAT. More details can be found at the following link: http://www.hmrc.gov.uk/working/intro/selfemployed.htm#2

Insurance

As a professional makeup artist you need to consider insurance to protect both you and your customers. Professional liability insurance also called professional indemnity insurance or errors and omissions in the USA is a form of liability insurance. This type of insurance helps protect professional advice and service providing individuals and businesses from bearing the full cost of defending themselves against a claim of negligence made by a client and any damages that may be awarded in a civil lawsuit.

Research the cost and coverage of liability insurance available in your area and decide on the best one for your business.

Advertising and Marketing Law

All businesses have a legal responsibility to ensure that any advertising claims are truthful and not misleading and that any marketing activity is within the law. Ensure that you read all relevant material to ensure that you follow the rules pertaining to:

- Truth in Advertising and Marketing Claims
- Telemarketing
- Data Protection
- Email Spam

Money

As with all businesses there are start-up costs involved; the costs of products, tools, supplies and the cost of transport. You'll also have on-going costs as you replace the skincare and makeup products and tools and supplies as they are used. Fortunately as a makeup artist you can start with a basic kit and build up your kit as you do business enabling you to offer more products and services to your customers as time goes on.

In addition you will have the expense of producing marketing materials. My key piece of advice if you are starting on small budget is to be very wise how you spend your money. As you see more and more clients you can build up your kit and spend more on advertising. To start with use free marketing tools at your disposal such as forum marketing online and word of mouth and networking in person offline.

Open up a separate business bank account so you can keep track of your spending on business expenses such as your kit and self-promotion.

Record Keeping

Create a file and keep receipts from all your business expenses and copies of all your invoices together. It helps to create monthly tabs or separate envelopes in the file and then at the end of every month calculate what money your business has made.

The difference between your sales and your costs is your profit. The money you have earned in your business. To calculate your profit add up all your business expense receipts and write that figure down and then add up all the money you received and write that down. Then take the money spent from the money received to find the money you have earned from your makeup artistry business that month.

At the end of 12 months you will then have 12 monthly totals that you can use to calculate your yearly expenses, sales (revenue) and money earned. If you prefer there are also accounting software packages that are geared to small businesses such as Quicken, Sage and QuickBooks.

Financial Forecast

Create a financial forecast to estimate what money you are expecting to come into your business in the form of sales and what expenses (costs) you have for the next few months.

The main advantage of a financial forecast is being able to track your actual sales and expenses against what you forecast them to be. It's particularly difficult when you start a business to know how much everything is going to cost, how many sales you will generate and how much money you'll make. A financial forecast helps to estimate how much money you need on a month to month basis to keep your business running.

After a few months you can look at the figures on your financial forecast and see which parts of your business are more successful and which parts are less successful. Which activities are generating you the most profit? If there is a particular activity in your business which is making you more money than any other decide whether you want to focus on that and become a specialist in that activity. By doing so you'll build up your reputation, be seen as an expert and consequently can charge higher prices.

For more information on other aspects of setting up and running a makeup artist business take a look at the resource section at the back of the book and visit our resource page at www.makemoneywithmakeup.com

Creating a Winning Beauty Portfolio that Showcases Your Skills to Prospective Employers and Clients

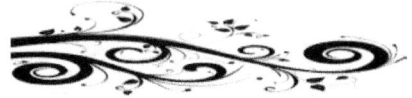

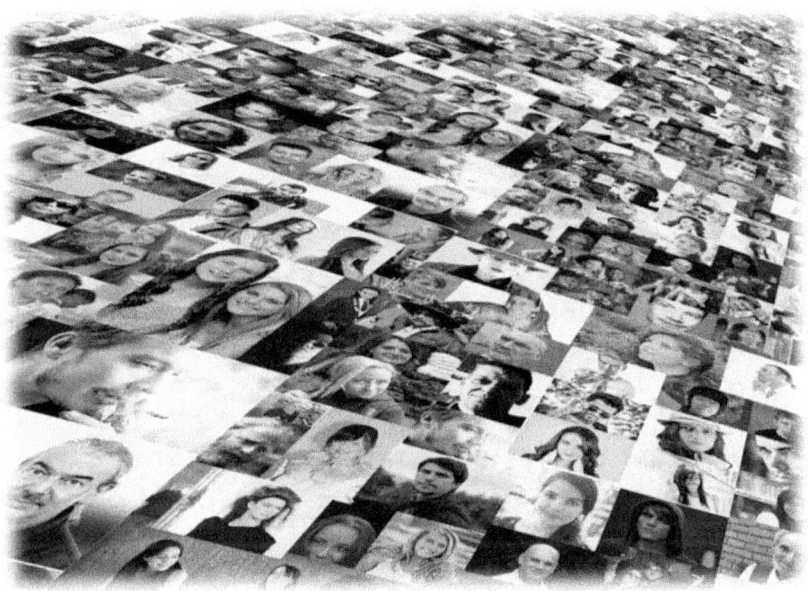

What is Portfolio?

A Portfolio is a collection of photos that showcase your skills and creativity as a Makeup Artist. You'll need it to show prospective clients what you can do for them. You can start with as few as 7-10 looks in your portfolio and build it up as you continue using your skills.

There are different types of portfolio ranging from a traditional display binder in a leather folder to an online graphical display. It is also possible these days to show your skills to the world by burning your before and after photographs to a CD, creating a downloadable MP4 of your work or building a slideshow of photos you can show on your website. You can even show the photos to prospective clients with a mobile device such as an ipad or Kindle.

Creating Your Beauty Portfolio

- **Take Lots of Photos**

It is never too late to start taking pictures for your portfolio. As soon as you start practising your skills you can take before and after photos of your work. Even at beauty school. This way you will also have a good record of how your skills progress over time.

You never know when you might be asked to do some work using your skills so it is always best to be prepared and have a portfolio of pictures even in the early days.

As soon as possible hire or barter with a professional photographer to ensure your photographs are of the highest quality. Often photographers are looking for makeup and hair professionals to create their own portfolios too!

A camera with high resolution and good lighting will help capture every detail of your work. The photographs should be taken up close, blocking out everything but face, hair and shoulders.

In addition, take a number of different photos at different angles to increase your chances of getting a quality shot. They should be eye- catching. The quality of the images in your portfolio will be a representation of you and the respect you have of your work. Don't downplay your talents by featuring grainy or blurry photos.

Take Before and After Photos

Take both before and after photos so you can showcase the transformation that your skills provide. As a makeup artist take a quick snapshot of your model with their hair up and no makeup and foundation and then take a photo afterwards with their hair down and looking fabulous to showcase the effects of a great make up job. You could

Get Your FREE Gift ...See Page 154

even ask the model not to smile in the before picture but to smile in the follow up one.

Find Models for Your Portfolio

You don't need years of experience to develop an impressive portfolio but you do need talent and models.

One place you can find makeup models is by volunteering at local fashion shows and photo shoots. Fashion shows employ many models so you can create a large collection of looks to add to your portfolio within a few hours. Try calling local modelling agencies and ask if they need photos of new talent.

You can also use your friends and family members to make a start on your portfolio too. The more people you can work with and practice your skills with the better.

Your portfolio should only contain your best work so make sure you make up a lot of models so you have more to choose from. In addition choose a selection of different models with different skin tones, hair colour, eye shape, face shape, age etc. You want to show that you can work with a variety of people to showcase your versatility. If you only show one type of model it will be assumed that that is all you can do!

Design Your Portfolio

To construct the more traditional beauty portfolio, you'll need to purchase a scrapbook or binder. Place each photo onto a heavy piece of black card. Use coloured pens and notes about each look to make your portfolio stand out.

Divide your portfolio into different sections with titles to show the different type of effect you are creating with your work. For example you could have a section for bridal hair and/or makeup, party hair and/or makeup, special effect hair and/or makeup, natural hair and/or makeup etc.

Make sure that your images are presented professionally in the portfolio. A leather bound portfolio will create a better impression than a plastic sleeve. Make sure your portfolio is always clean and professional looking.

The traditional black leather binder is 11" by 14" or 12" by 15" with photos of at least 8.5" by 11" or bigger to show details of the makeup.

- **Include the following in Your Portfolio?**
    - o Before and after photos
    - o Testimonials from satisfied customers (letters or emails for example)
    - o Copies of Press Releases regarding your business

- A brochure and/or business cards
- Letters of recommendation

- **Feature Only your Best Work**

Your portfolio should only contain your best work so make sure you make up a lot of models so you have more to choose from. In addition choose a selection of different models with different skin tones, hair colour, eye shape, face shape, age etc. You want to show that you can work with a variety of people to showcase your versatility. If you only show one type of model it will be assumed that that is all you can do! Only choose images of your work that you're truly proud of. If that means that in the beginning you only have three images in your portfolio, that's absolutely fine. Featuring fewer but high quality images and showcasing high quality work will be better than featuring more work of less quality. You do not want to give any reason for potential clients to question your abilities.

- **Include the Type of Work You're Interested in Doing**

It is up to you what you put in your portfolio so focus primarily on showcasing those skills that you like to do most of all. For example if you like bridal work put more images of bridal work in your portfolio and minimize any other type of work. You'll attract potential clients who are interested in the look you show the most.

- **Keep Your Portfolio Updated**

In the beauty industry styles and trends are constantly changing so it is important that your portfolio stays up to date with all these changes too. Clients always 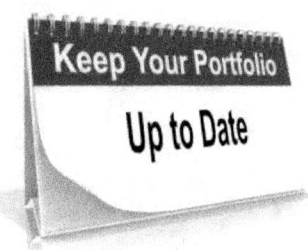 want to be reassured their makeup artist or stylist can create any style they request. The best reassurance for them will always be an up-to-date portfolio of your best work. Be seen as the professional you are.

- **Include a Brief Background Story with Each Image**

Make the portfolio even more interesting by including a short paragraph with each image. Explain what techniques you used to get that particular look. Get permission from your clients to showcase their completed look and add a brief testimonial.

Types of Beauty Portfolio

There are Four Types of Beauty Portfolios to help you showcase your talents as a beauty professional and show prospective employers and clients.

Traditional Portfolio

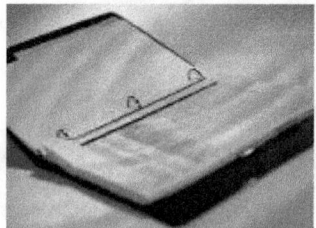

Traditional portfolios are bound in display binders but go ahead and use your creativity to design one unique to you.

Specialist Portfolio

The specialist beauty portfolio is suitable if you specialize in a certain type of work. For example if you specialize in bridal makeup or hair then put together a bridal portfolio showcasing just the work you've done with brides. If you are seeking work with special effects or theatre work for example create portfolios specifically to showcase this type of makeup artistry and/or hair creations.

If you're seeking work in film, TV or fashion make sure your portfolio is of a professional quality. Your photos also need to reflect what's currently in fashion as well as classical looks. They must not look outdated as that will reflect poorly on you. You'll need to also focus on the quality of the camera as you must avoid showing amateurish photographs.

- **Video Portfolio**

In addition to specialist portfolios you may want to consider a video portfolio comprised of your photos and information. You can add such videos to video sharing sites 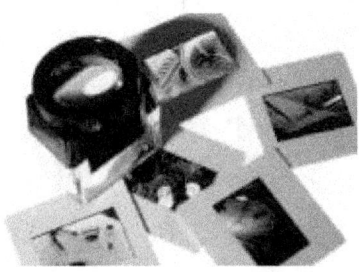 online, create an MP4 or burn to a CD to share with others.

Online Portfolio

When you put your portfolio online, your work becomes more accessible and more available to potential employers. You can add graphics or a video and use it to showcase your skills on various platforms online.

In addition you can create a website. Make sure your homepage is eye- catching and that the site includes a photo gallery with high-quality images and short descriptions.

Use Hi-Res Images on your website. Poor quality photos reflect poorly on your work. You want your images to reflect the high standard of your work.

For those of you who don't have a website visit (http://makemoneywithmakeup.com) for more details on how to get one created for you. One especially designed for showcasing your work as a makeup artist.

In summary one of the most important items to have as a Makeup Artist is a quality portfolio. Make sure you get into the habit of taking before and after photos and updating your portfolio with the photos that show your talent at its best.

When visiting prospective customers with your portfolio it's a good idea to include your brochure, testimonials from satisfied customers, letters of recommendation, any press coverage of your business and photographs of you working with clients.

For more information on creating a portfolio take a look at the resource section at the back of the book and visit our resource page at makemoneywithmakeup.com

A strong brow, bedroom eyes, a bump on the nose – these are the features that inspire me. Beauty isn't about looking perfect. It's about celebrating your individuality   *Bobbi Brown*

The Makeup of Makeup Artists: What to Choose

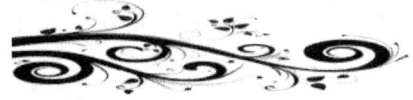

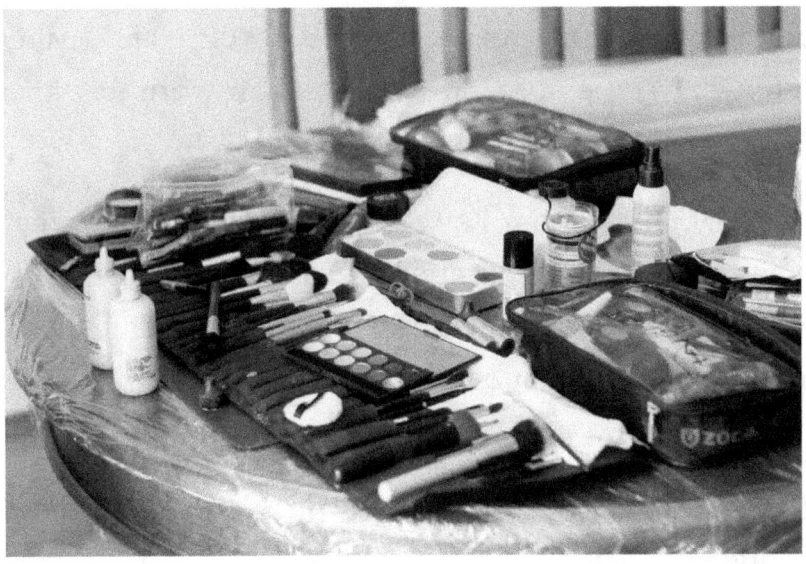

There are hundreds of brands of makeup to choose from out there on the market today. In this chapter we're going to look at Makeup.

The brands of Makeup you choose will depend on price, the type of makeup artistry that you do and personal preference. Makeup artists usually have a preferred company for different products they use. It is important to take care to choose products that work well together though.

At the beginning it's a good idea to join a cosmetics company. Doing so is a great way to get discounted makeup that you can use in your business. Look for quality though. Your clients expect great results and using makeup that comes off too quickly when worn will give you a bad reputation! Not what you want!

I personally chose Mary Kay. In addition to getting great training on makeup application I had a 40% discount on the cosmetics I used in my business and my clients loved the quality of the makeup too.

Today we are going to look at the types of makeup that a makeup artist needs to include in their kit and a description of each.

First of all let's take a look at some Makeup Terminology to make sure we understand the different types of makeup available today.

Makeup Terminology

Cosmetics: beauty products that can be applied to the face, hands and body

Makeup: beauty products designed specifically for the face

Natural Makeup: Designed for everyday wear

Character Makeup: Designed specifically for characters in TV, film video and theatre work. It may be used to make actors look older, younger, rich, poor, ill, injured, alien etc.,

Stage Makeup: Makeup designed for actors or other performers on stage, where lighting creates special challenges

Special Effects Makeup: As the name implies makeup required for special effects

Fashion Makeup: Makeup specifically designed for models showcasing fashion

Glamour Makeup: Special event Makeup designed to make a person look fabulous for an event

Corrective Makeup: Makeup specially created to cover or camouflage scars, burns, skin problems or physical disfigurements.

Airbrush makeup: Makeup sprayed onto the skin using an airbrush

Get Your FREE Gift ...See Page 154

HD Makeup: A technique used to make up the face for HD cameras

Mineral Makeup: Makeup made up of minerals such as iron oxides, talc, zinc oxide and titanium dioxide that are ground and milled or broken into very tiny particles.

Makeup Artist: Anyone who applies makeup professionally

Types of Makeup

Foundation

The right foundation provides a smooth, flawless base for colour. It is the most important part of any makeup application.

So what makes it right?

Choosing a foundation

It is best to use natural daylight when choosing a foundation colour. The shade should be tried along your jaw line rather than on the back of the hand, which is a different shade to your facial skin tone. If the foundation blends in completely so it is hardly visible it is the right shade for you.

Foundation is extremely noticeable when applied in the wrong shade or not properly blended. Do avoid the orange line at the edge of the face and do not try to alter your skin colour/tone by using a darker shade which can be very aging and a lighter one that can make you look unwell. Colour can be added later with bronzers and blushers.

Bronze skin tones come in more than 35 variation of colour compared to about 10 for ivory skin so bronze skin tones may need to customize their foundation by mixing two shades together for the best match.

Foundation is designed to provide an even skin tone, cover blemishes and protect the skin. Not be noticeable for everyone to see. Some foundations have additional benefits such as sun protection (SPF), added vitamins and light reflecting particles.

Concealer

Concealer serves two functions: either to camouflage or to highlight. It usually comes in small containers and is only used sparingly on the face.

Coloured concealer can be used to counterbalance discolouration on fairer skin tones. Red can be neutralized by green, pink by pale yellow and rosy by pale lilac.

To apply dab a small amount on what you're trying to hide and blend in. Be careful to use a colour that is not too light, which will have the opposite effect and draw attention to the area.

To hide dark under eye circles choose a concealer that is one shade lighter than your foundation, dab onto the dark circle and blend outwards into the foundation application. Dab foundation over the top of the concealer. Blending is key.

Blusher

Blusher adds colour and vitality to the face, giving definition where there was none. Blushers come into many different colours and tones – the most common being pink, peach, purple and brown tones. Most blushers are now in powder form but you can still use cream blushers underneath foundation. Powder blush is more easily blended and can create a more natural look.

Face Powders

A good face powder should be easy to apply, be smooth on the skin and allow the colour of the foundation to be seen without changing the base colour. The main component of powder is talc which gives slip, translucency and covering power. Used to set foundation, control shine and finish a makeup look once applied to protect from heat and perspiration.

Eye Shadows

The purpose of eye shadow is to accentuate the eyes and make them look brighter, to coordinate the face with an overall look, and to complement or contrast the natural eye colour. It comes in nearly every colour and finish from matte to shiny. You'll need a range of colours to choose from.

Eye Liner

Eyeliner is available in cake, liquid and pencil form. It is used to define the shape of the eye and give the appearance of opening them up. Depending on the effect desired it is placed on the top, bottom or both lids and either encircles the entire eye or is used on the outer edges only. Softer liners such as cake or pencil can be smudged using a sponge tipped applicator or a cotton bud giving a softer definition to the eye.

Eyebrow Pencils

Eyebrow pencils are used to add definition to the eyebrow area as well as balancing and infilling missing areas of eyebrow. They come in various colours including grey, brown, blonde and black.

Get Your FREE Gift ...See Page 154

To apply brush the brows into shape then use light feather strokes on the brow hair itself to define them. Brush through after application.

Mascara

Mascara is used to give definition to the eyes by thickening, lengthening and darkening the lashes. The most popular is the liquid mascara. Mascara comes in a selection of black, brown, and a variety of fashion colours.

Formulations

- Waterproof
- Smudge proof
- Lash Lengthening
- Protein Enriched
- Thickening

Safety tip: Do not pump the wand in and out of the mascara tube as you are pumping in air which results in it drying out quicker and can introduce bacteria potentially leading to eye infections.

Lipsticks

Coming in a vast array of pots, wands, sticks and pencils in a wide assortment of colours lipsticks are used to define, enhance and balance lip shape. A lipstick should be chosen to enhance the makeup and reflect the colour of the clothes that are being worn

Lip Gloss

Gloss can be clear or pigmented and used under or over lipstick or on its own depending on the effect required (semi-shine or full on shine) Glosses are not as durable as lipsticks and need reapplying. They come in wands or pots and are used to add sheen and sparkle to the lips after or instead of the application of lip colour.

Lip Liners and Pencils

These are used to outline the lips. Pencils are good for correcting the lip area by balancing or realigning the lips. They also help in stopping the 'bleeding' effect around the mouth

You can spend a lot of money on purchasing the tools, and supplies you'll need as a makeup artist so it's advisable to build your supplies up bit by bit as the jobs come in. You don't need everything when you first start (however tempting it all is). You need just enough to cover each assignment as it comes along. As the money comes in by all means invest it into purchasing more tools and supplies for the business but watch your costs at the beginning if money is an issue.

For more information on where to get makeup take a look at the resource section at the back of the book and visit our resource page at makemoneywithmakeup.com

Let's take a look at what supplies and tools to include in your Makeup Artist Kit.

Makeup is a way for a woman to look and feel like herself, only prettier and more confident.

Bobbi Brown

Makeup Artist Supplies

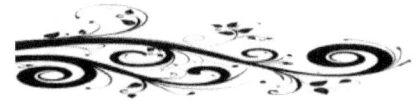

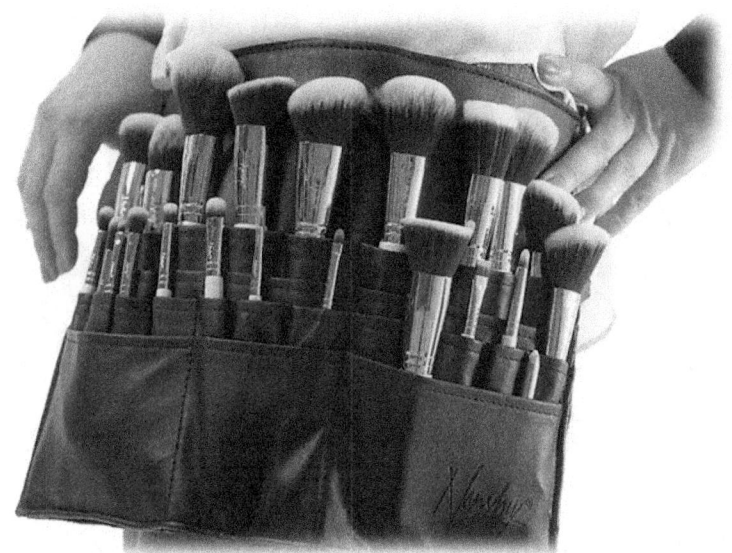

Makeup Artist Bag

Every makeup artist needs a bag, case or something to hold their tools and supplies. Over time as you accumulate more tools and supplies you'll probably need to invest in larger bags, cases or have specific ones for different jobs: One for bridal makeup, one for stage makeup, one for live events for examples.

You might want to invest in an aluminium case (also known as train cases) with lots of compartments to put

Get Your FREE Gift ...See Page 154

items in. You can also get huge pull along suitcases or smaller cases with wheels for mobility.

Just think what jobs you have or might have coming up when deciding on what to purchase. You may have to carry bags a long way, upstairs, outside etc., depending on your location. From my experience the weight of the case when empty is an important consideration: the lighter the better. Check that the handles and hinges are suitable for heavy usage too.

For quick access to different products in various drawers and compartments of your makeup artist bag add some tape and label the different types of products e.g.) lip colours, eye colours, foundations.

If your assignments change a lot you might want to think about getting one case that can be wheeled around and another smaller one that can be carried.

Makeup Artist Set Bags

A Makeup Artist Set Bag is useful for the working Artist on the set. They allow you to carry the essential items needed for touch-ups. It's helpful if the set bag has lots of compartments. They are usually made of leather, canvas or clear plastic with lots of pockets to hold things like brushes, sponges and product.

For more examples of makeup bags and cases an online search will reveal lots of options.

Makeup Apron

A Must Have for the Makeup Artist on the Set. Multiple pockets, pouches and hooks for Brushes, Tools, Mobile Phone or other personal items.

Brush and Tool Belt

It holds all the important tools of the trade such as makeup brushes, powder brushes, eyebrow pencils, scissors, combs, and more. A brush and tool belt is a great way to keep your supplies close at hand.

Makeup Artist Tools

Makeup Tools such as brushes, sponges, applicators and other gadgets are essential to the work of the Makeup Artist and investment in this area is often the key to their success. With the right tools a good makeup artist can use almost any brand of makeup. The Key tools are: brushes, cosmetic sponges, mixing palettes, tweezers, spatulas, sharpeners, eyelash curlers, cue tips (swabs), cotton wool, disposable makeup applicators and tissues.

Expect to spend a bit of money on good quality brushes. Essential if you want to do a quality makeover on a client!

Make sure you monitor your supplies and check your bags after every assignment and replace what's running low. There's nothing worse than running out of an essential item on the job itself. Spending time after each assignment to restock your kit is advantageous since new jobs can come up sometimes at the last minute. Be ready for them!

Makeup Kit Checklist
Cleanser, Freshener, Moisturizer

Eye Makeup Remover

Blotting Tissues

Lip mask and balm

Foundation (various shades and light, medium, and heavy coverage, also mineral powder of various shades)

Both Light and Heavier "camouflage" concealer in various shades

Get Your FREE Gift ...See Page 154

Blusher in pinks, peaches and reds

Eye shadows (look for palettes or create your own)

Eyeliners in a range of shades including black, brown and white

Eyebrow pencils in black, brown and blonde

Lip colours including reds, pinks, peaches and browns

Lip pencils to complement lip colours

Lip gloss in clear and a variety of finishes (sparkling, tinted, metallic, etc.)

Loose powder in light to dark and translucent

Mascara in black and brown-black

Brushes (at least two of each):

Powder brush

Blush brush

Sponge brush

Blending brush

Contour brush

Eyeliner brush

Angled eyebrow brush

Lip brush

Concealer brush

Eye shadow brush

Detail brush

Foundation Brushes:

Mineral

Liquid

Sponges: cosmetic wedges

Cotton wool

False eyelash strips and clusters, and application glues for each type

Eyelash curler

Makeup pencil sharpener

Tweezers

Scissors

Tissues

Hand Cleaner

Cue tips (swabs)

Disposable applicators (eye shadow, lip brushes and mascara wands)

Anti-shine (e.g. Neutrogena shine control gel or Super Matte Anti-Shine)

A makeup cape

Paper towels

Quick drying cosmetic brush cleaner

Hair clips

You may also want to add:

Makeup palette and spatula (for mixing foundations or lip colours)

Spray bottle with water

Small bowl for water to dip sponges or brushes into

Hip apron to carry cosmetics on set

A small portable chair for you to sit on for long waits out

on location

A portable professional lighted mirror station

A tall makeup chair (makes your job as a makeup artist much easier as you don't have to bend as much)

Set Bag Checklist

Use this checklist to make sure you have the necessary supplies to do any on-set touchups needed. You can add to or customize this list as you see fit.

Blush

Eyeshadow palette

Hairbrush

Comb

Blotting paper

Travel-size hairspray

A few brushes

A few sponges

Lipstick palette

Lip gloss

Foundation in a few shades

Tissues

A cosmetic puff

Pressed powder

Other:

For more information on where to get makeup supplies take a look at the resource section at the back of the book and visit our resource page at makemoneywithmakeup.com

Introduction to Health and Safety

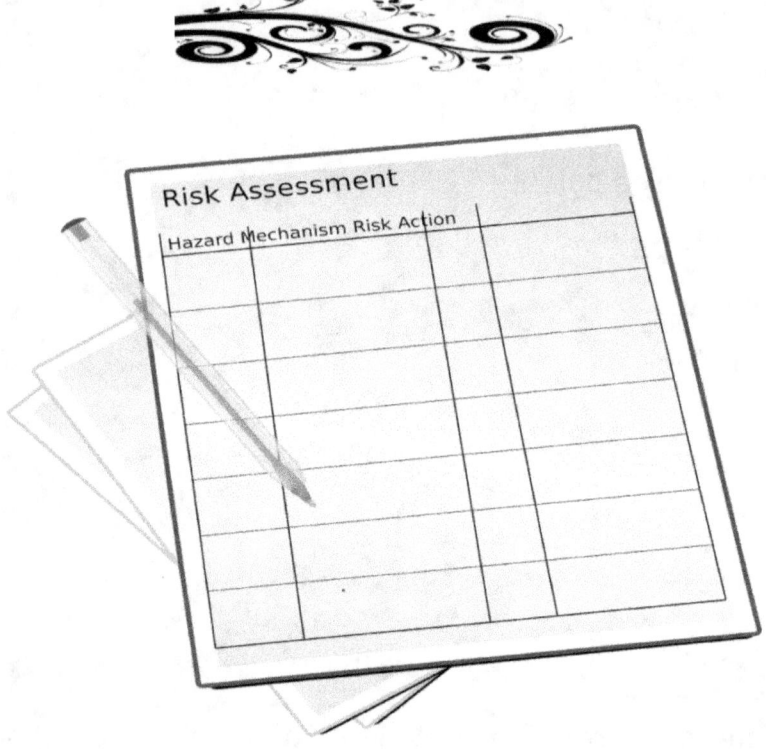

Maintaining a very high standard of hygiene and cleanliness is essential to your makeup artistry business. As a Professional Makeup Artist you want to ensure that you follow health and safety guidelines in everything you do to safeguard your own and others' health. Let's take a look at the ways to keep you and your customers safe.

Tips for Keeping You and Your Customers Safe

Personal Hygiene

As a makeup artist you will be working in close proximity to others. Perspiration, smoking, strong and spicy foods and other things that could cause unpleasant odours should be avoided to help everyone work comfortably together.

In addition, the effort you put into getting ready to go out and the way you present yourself says a lot about you and will affect the way people react to you.

Your personal hygiene must be impeccable: Well-groomed with clean hair and nails and a light touch of makeup.

When you are working on other people keep your hair away from them. If it is long it's a good idea to tie it back.

A uniform helps you look more professional. Make sure it is clean at all times.

Don't forget to wash your hands! It is important to wash them frequently and in front of the client.

Get Your FREE Gift ...See Page 154

Think about the impression you give to your clients. Ask yourself if you would accept a makeover from someone looking like you!

Tools, Products and Supplies

Everything you use must be clean before you use it; Towels, headbands, tools, work area products and more. If these are not clean then you run the risk of infecting yourself and whoever uses your equipment or products.

This is especially true for makeup so be aware of sharing makeup with your friends. You do not know if you could be causing an eye infection, such as conjunctivitis, to be transmitted to your friend or vice versa.

- All work surfaces and trolleys should be disinfected daily
- New towels should be used for each client
- Reusable tools need to be sterilized after every treatment

It's even better to sanitize, clean and wipe all tools and products in front of your client to make sure they know you are hygienic and follow health and safety precautions and procedures.

Make sure your brushes are kept clean. On the job you can use a brush cleaner between clients. Even when your brushes are clean, it's a good idea to use a mist cleaner and lightly clean brushes in front of your client. Let your client know that her comfort is important to you.

No double dipping! Use a fresh brush or applicator when getting extra product for the same client to avoid contaminating your cosmetic supplies.

For other products where a disposable wand or similar tool isn't convenient, simply scoop out the amount of product you need and place it on a painter's palette, paper towel or small tray (whatever is handy as long as it's clean.)

When working with a client, use a spatula to place lipstick or gloss on a palette and apply with a lip brush.

Sanitize makeup pencils by sharpening them between clients. Do not forget to clean your sharpener each time too.

Use latex-free sponges to avoid potential allergic reactions. Always ask your client if they have any allergies or sensitivities.

Don't blow on the product, brushes or client's face. It's as bad as spitting on them. It is unsanitary and unprofessional. Always tap off excess powder on your brushes and use cotton wool or something similar to remove powder from trays.

Make sure you clean everything between clients

Be aware of infections and that you do not spread them. Cross infection can be caused by direct contact or indirect contact.

Direct contact with another person by touching an infected area of a person's skin or by inhaling airborne droplets ejected from the nose or mouth when an infected person is speaking, coughing or sneezing.

Indirect contact with an infected article is a less obvious method of infection. It involves the passing of infection from a person to an object for example a towel, jar of cream and then transferring the infection from the object to a second person. The two people may never meet having used the towel or pot of cream at different times.

Use disposable applicators

If at any point in time you or a client develops an eye infection like conjunctivitis or pink eye, you should immediately throw away any makeup that has come in contact with the eyes and just start fresh with new products.

Use isopropyl alcohol of 90% or greater to sanitize any tools including tweezers, scissors and lash curlers. Be sure the alcohol has evaporated before using the tool on the client.

Reshape small, fluffy brushes (like eye shadow brushes) into their proper form while they are still moist, so when they dry, they are like new.

Pots and tubes must be kept clean as dirt provides food for bacteria. Make sure the tops are not cracked or broken since this allows the bacteria in to contaminate the product.

Do not put your fingers into the pots

Take care when disposing of waste

Cosmetics Freshness Chart

The following table is a guide to how long to keep each type of make up before they should be disposed of.

Powders	8 – 12 months
Eye Liners	3 – 6 months
Eye Shadows	3 – 12 months
Mascara	3 months
Concealer	4 – 6 months
Lipstick	12 months

Professional Services to Offer Your Clients: Mini Facials

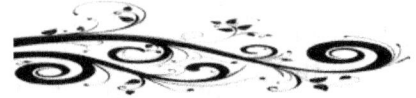

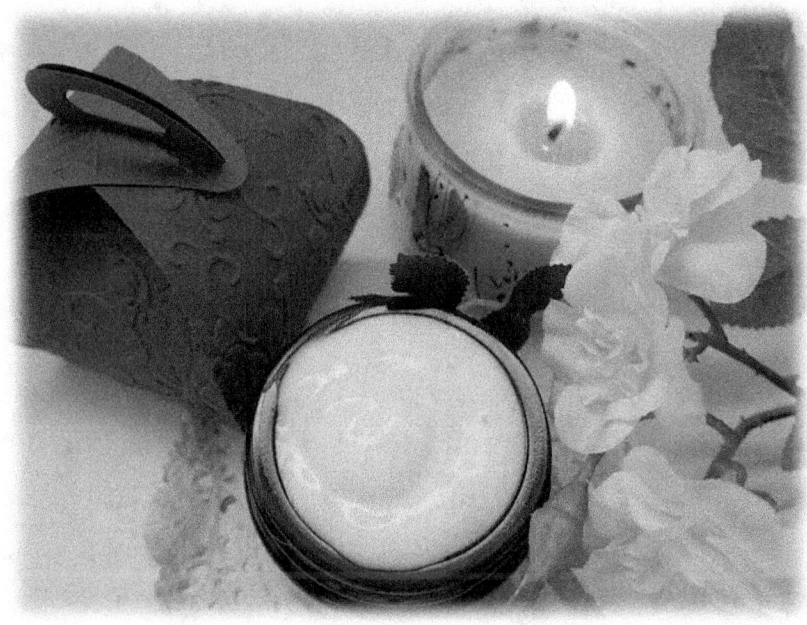

As a makeup artist you have the opportunity to educate your clients about skincare as well as makeup application. You can offer mini facials as well as classes and demonstrations to show the optimum way for people to look after their skin. It is often said that makeup is only as good as the skin underneath. From my experience as a makeup artist I can tell you that it is a lot easier to create a great makeover when the skin underneath is well looked after.

In this chapter we are going to be looking at how to take care of your skin, different skin types, how to prepare your skin for makeup and looking at how skin ages in order that you have the knowledge necessary to answer your client's questions. Then we'll detail a step by step mini facial you can do for a client.

Prepare Your Skin for Makeup

Makeup is only as good as the skin underneath it. Many products exist which attempt to disguise imperfection but it is difficult for makeup to look good if the skin underneath is in poor condition. In addition, many people complain that their makeup seems to disappear after just a few hours. The cosmetic products on the market today are designed to last until they are removed at night so it's often improper skin preparation that causes it to disappear. Therefore, let's spend a bit of time looking at our skin and how we can keep it in optimum condition before we move on to applying makeup.

Our Skin

Our skin protects us from the ravages of everyday living. It protects us from ultra-violet light, pollution, the weather (extremes of hot and cold), wind and sun, and central heating. We need to take care of it!

A beautiful skin is a healthy balanced skin. We can protect it by:

- Eating a balanced diet – plenty of vegetables, fruit and fibre. Foods containing vitamins A, B and C, proteins and essential fatty acids.
- Drinking plenty of water
- Getting enough sleep (on average 6 – 8 hours per night)
- Protecting the skin and keeping it clean (using a good skincare range which we'll talk about in a minute)
- Avoiding harsh treatment (be careful what products you use on your skin)
- Exercising regularly
- Not smoking (which causes oxygen and vitamin C depletion in the skin cells – both of which are needed for healthy skin)
- Controlling alcohol intake (alcohol raises the blood pressure and causes the blood capillaries to rupture causing permanent damage. It dehydrates the skin and long term can cause puffiness, coarsening of

the skin texture, premature aging and rending of the skin)

Skincare: 3 Simple Steps to Better Skin

There are three very simple, basic steps that take just a couple of minutes before you begin your makeup application.

1. Cleanse

The first step is to cleanse the skin. There are different cleansers on the market but a good cleanser will:

Remove makeup, dirt and grime effectively

Be easily applied and removed

Types of Cleanser

Creams

o   ideal for mature skins and dry skin types

o   They dissolve the pigmented waxes found in make-up

o   They have a cooling effect on the skin

o   They are easily removed

Milks

o Light in Consistency

o Not effective in removing heavy – makeup

Lotions

o Useful on congested or oily skins

o Leave very little residue on the skin after removal

o Can be very strong

Soapless cleansers and bars

o For those who prefer the feel of soap but not it's drying effect

o Ph balanced

o Effective on oily and acne prone skin

Cleansing wipes

o Often used to save time

o Come with or without the need to dampen them

Beware the fragrances in some if you have sensitive skin

3 in 1 products

o Contain cleanser, toner and exfoliant

o Designed to save time and can be very effective

Be careful using on sensitive skin and skin prone to blemishes

Application

The cleanser should be gently applied to the surface of the skin in an upward and outward movement and then removed (with a warm wet cloth or cotton pads) and rinsed off with tepid water. Use a specially designed product for the eye area since this area is very fragile.

2. Toners and Exfoliators

This is used after you have cleansed your skin. It removes any remaining product on the skin leaving it feeling clean and fresh and prepared for an application of moisturiser.

Exfoliators

Exfoliators or masks are designed to help get rid of dead skin cells on the surface of the face. They smooth the skin surface, stimulate the blood and lymphatic flow, helping in the elimination of waste products. All skin types benefit from using exfoliating products. There are 2 main types: peeling creams and pore grains or facial scrubs.

Masking the Face

Beneficial Effects of Masks:

Sooth and calm

Soften

Exfoliate

Moisturize

Deep Cleanse

Remove excess oil

Stimulate circulation

Rejuvenate

Refresh

Revitalize

Clean pores

Types of Masks

Facial masks are formulated according to skin type. Clay and mud masks are suitable for oily skin and cream-based masks for dry skin

Setting: These masks are clay based , dry on the skin and are peeled off

Non Setting: These are biological and clay-based to which oil has been added. They are cooling and soothing on the skin but do not set and can be washed off.

Specialized Masks such as honey, paraffin wax, oil, gel, thermal and cream. All serve different purposes.

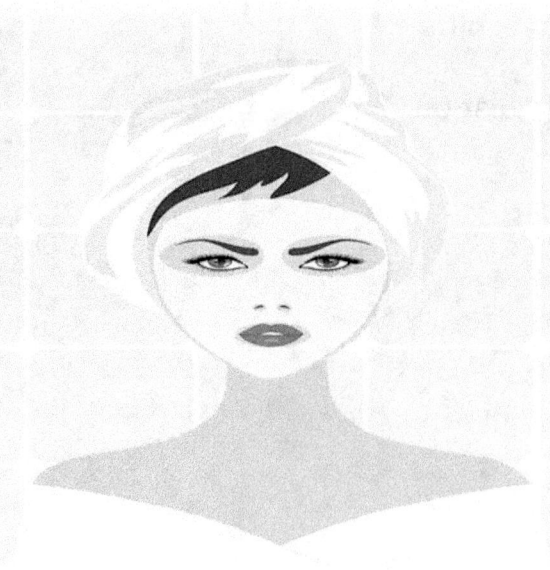

Applying a Mask

A mask should be applied after cleansing and before the toner.

They can be applied using a brush, spatula or very clean hands

They must be applied evenly or they can evaporate too quickly giving a burning or itching sensation on the skin

If there is any feeling of discomfort remove immediately

Apply starting at the base of the neck and work up the face – using the same procedure as in cleansing

Be careful to avoid the hairline, eyes, mouth and nostrils

Once the masks has dried or had its allotted time it should be removed with warm water and sponges, cotton wool pads, or a clean, soft flannel. Once all traces of the mask have been removed the skin should feel clean and refreshed.

3. Moisturisers

Moisturizing is an important step that helps retain the natural moisture in your skin and prevents your makeup from entering your pores. If your makeup doesn't recede into your pores then it will remain on the surface of the skin where it belongs, therefore lasting much longer. Make sure to begin with a freshly washed face, and then apply your moisturiser. Moisturiser evens the skin's porosity and works best when left to absorb for a few minutes before you apply your makeup. You can choose a light moisturizer or a heavy one; just choose the right one for your particular skin type.

Moisturisers for normal skin are usually light to help even out any dry areas

Moisturisers for dry skin are usually higher in emollients and are richer

Moisturisers for sensitive skin are fragrance and irritant-free

Moisturisers for oily skin are extremely light and don't clog pores. Many have oil absorbing properties in them that help control the oil. Oily skin needs moisturizer because it can often be over-dried by cleansers. This results in the complexion appearing even greasier.

After you have consistently practiced this routine for a few months you will not only notice a great difference in your make-up but will also begin to enjoy a much finer complexion

Get Your FREE Gift ...See Page 154

What is your Skin Type?

When choosing skin care products it is important to know your skin type to look after it properly.

Adapted from Making Aromatherapy Creams and Lotions, by Donna Marie (Storey Books, 2000).

This great little quiz will help identify yours

1. Does your skin look dull or flaky?

2. Does your skin have a shiny, slippery texture?

3. Does your skin feel itchy and taut?

4. Do you have enlarged or clogged pores, or acne?

5. Does your skin react adversely to cosmetics containing alcohol, synthetics, fragrances, and artificial colors?

6. Does your skin appear consistently plump, moist, and vibrant?

7. Does your forehead, nose, or chin appear oily, while the skin around your cheeks, eyes, and mouth is normal or dry?

If you answered yes to 1 or 3, you have DRY skin.
If you answered yes to 2 or 4, you have OILY skin.

Get Your FREE Gift ...See Page 154

If you answered yes to 5, you have SENSITIVE skin.

If you answered yes to 6, you have NORMAL skin.

If you answered yes to 7, you have COMBINATION skin.

Dry Skin

Dry skin is prone to aging quickly.

Features include:

• A flaky and taut appearance

• Fine texture, often with fine lining

• A fragile, transparent tone with vascular appearance on the cheeks

• Often increased colour and responds quickly to stimulation

• Possibly, irritated sensitive areas

• Rarely any spots

• Exposure to wind and cold will cause fine lines to develop quickly around eyes and mouth

• Dilated capillaries causing flushed areas

It needs lots of moisture and protection so it is important to drink lots of water and use products that contain a balanced combination of oil and water to soothe and hydrate the skin

Oily Skin

Oily skin ages more slowly than dry skin and remains younger looking and more supple over time. It still has a tendency to dryness as it gets older.

Features include:

- A slight shine
- Open pores and a coarse texture
- Few, if any, lines
- A sallow tone
- Prone to spots and blemishes
- Quickly develops shine and does not hold makeup well
- Excellent conditions for bacterial growth

This skin type needs to be cleaned and exfoliated gently but effectively to keep it looking smooth and spot free. Be wary of products that are too harsh which will only make blemishes worse.

Sensitive Skin

Sensitive skin needs gentle, natural products to keep it in optimum condition.

Features include:

- Sometimes a vascular appearance with dilated capillaries

• Flushed areas and patchy colouring

• Reacts quickly, producing an erythema (redness of the skin), in response to pressure, heat, abrasion or products.

• Prone to allergic reaction (causing dehydration and fine lines)

• Reacts particularly to spirit based or heavily perfumed products

Normal Skin

The normal skin type is very rare and usually found in pre-adolescents.

Features include:

• No shine
• No flaky patches
• A fine, even texture
• Clear bright tone
• Rare, if any, lines
• Rare, if any, spots or blemishes

A balanced skincare routine and protection will keep it looking good for longer.

Combination Skin

Combination Skin has an oily centre panel (T panel) and normal or dry cheeks.

Features include:

May include one or other of the following alongside a mixture, 'combination' of the other skin types:
• greasy nose and chin with shine and blemishes
• dry forehead with fine lining
• dry cheeks with vascular appearance
• normal skin on neck

Use gentle but effective products that will clean and exfoliate the T panel and provide moisture and protection for the cheeks.

How Skin Ages

Skin becomes Drier

Sebum production slows down and because there's also a decrease in the number of sweat glands, sweat production declines. Together these changes translate into drier skin. An appropriate basic skincare program will help alleviate the tightness, reduce the flakiness, and soften and protect dry skin.

Get Your FREE Gift ...See Page 154

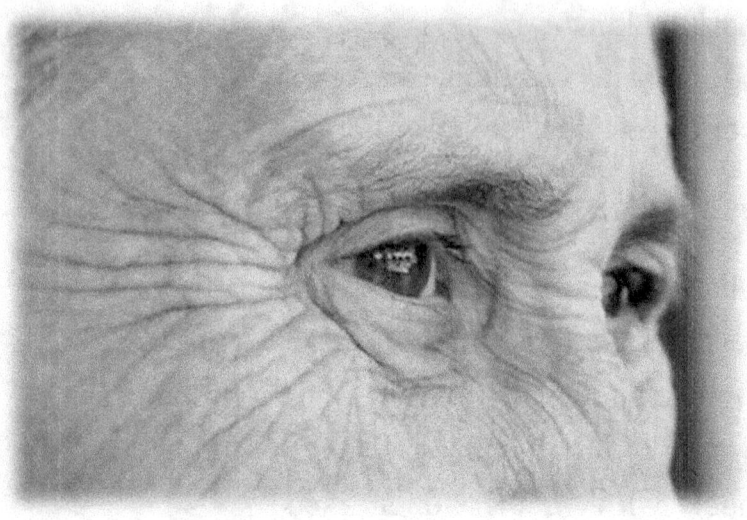

The skin becomes less flexible

The dermis also becomes less flexible. As skin ages, the structure of elastin and collagen fibers tends to change – a process that results in the loss of resilience and elasticity.

Wrinkling

Still another part of the aging process is wrinkling. Wrinkles tend to form first around the outside comers of the eyes, between the brows and near the mouth – along the lip line, and smile lines that extend from the outside comers of the mouth up to the sides of the nose. This area

Get Your FREE Gift …See Page 154

of your facial skin is stretched repeatedly when you smile, laugh and frown so the more animated your facial expressions, the earlier in life the wrinkles could form.

Droopy Skin

The loss of fatty pads is another problem. As skin ages, some of the underlying fatty tissue is loss. At first, the fat loss is flattering because it draws attention to facial contours, particularly the cheekbones. However, once coupled with the loss of elasticity, droopy skin may not be far behind. The skin across the cheeks may sag, the nose may appear longer and jowls may form.

More prone to skin damage

As skin ages, there's also a decrease in the number of melanocytes – the cells that produce the pigment that gives skin its colour. The decrease in these cells causes the skin to become lighter as well as more vulnerable to damage from the sun.

How to do a Mini Facial

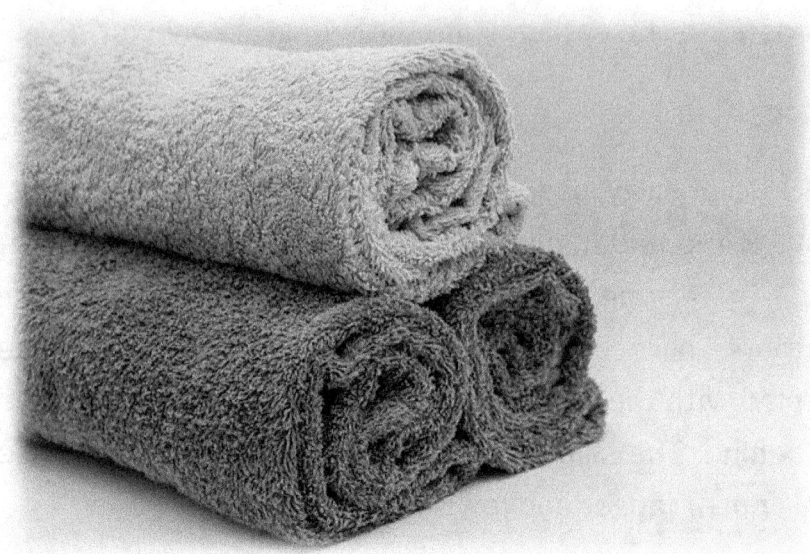

What you need:

Access to water

Low lighting /candles, music to create a relaxing atmosphere

Head band

Towel

Damp cotton wool pads, squares, sponges or a soft , clean flannel

Cleaner, toner and moisturiser suitable to your skin type

Get Your FREE Gift ...See Page 154

Eye makeup remover

Mask suitable to your skin type

Eye cream

Steps to follow

1 Wash your hands

2 Clean the face and neck by following the cleansing routine

The cleanser should be gently applied to the surface of the skin in an upward and outward movement and then removed (with a warm wet cloth or cotton pads) and rinsed off with tepid water. Use a specially designed product for the eye area since this area is very fragile.

3 Lie down, place small, wet, warm towel on the face and relax. Leave it on until it becomes almost cold.

4 Rinse the towel in warm water

5 Apply the mask and lie down again. Leave the mask on for the recommended time.

6 Take off the mask with warm water and clean the skin with the towel

7 Apply toner with damp cotton wool.

Get Your FREE Gift ...See Page 154

8 Apply eye cream

9   Apply moisturiser to neck and face

10 Blot with tissue

Understanding all about skin and how to take care of it enables you to be a better makeup artist. Your clients will expect you to know all about what type of skin they have and how to look after it. They look to you as the expert and by providing them the answers they seek you are seen as the professional that you are.

Professional Services to Offer Your Clients: Makeup Application

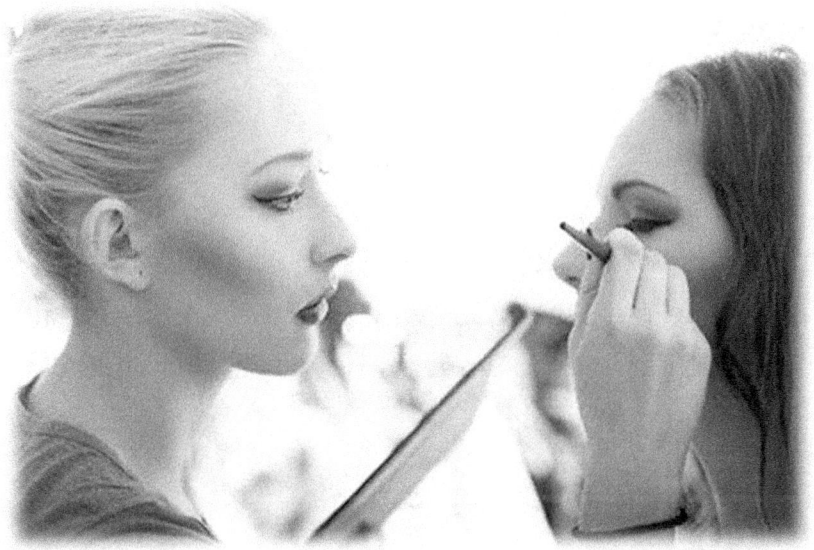

Makeup Application: the main reason why makeup artists become makeup artists. It gives you the chance to be creative and it's a great feeling when you transform someone before their eyes and they love the finished result.

In this chapter we are going to be looking at how to choose the right foundation, the different types of

Get Your FREE Gift ...See Page 154

foundation, how to apply foundation, concealer, face powder, highlighter and blusher and how to apply products to the eye area and lips.

Applying makeup should be viewed like an artist with basic rules to follow. We start with the canvas prepared by cleansing then the wash is applied (foundation). Next it is on to colour, shading and highlighting to produce the finished painting.

Makeup should be fun and suit the personality of the person and the occasion. You should never be afraid to experiment with colour as this is the only way you are going to find out what goes with what. There are no firm rules only guidelines to work by. However, such guidelines are a good starting point.

Basic Order of Makeup Application

Foundation and Concealer

Face Powder

Blusher

Eye Makeup: Eye Shadow, Eye Liner, Brow Pencil (if needed),

Mascara

Lip Pencil

Lipstick and Lip Gloss

Choosing the Right Foundation for Your Skin

It is best to use natural daylight when choosing a foundation colour. The shade should be tried along your jaw line rather than on the back of the hand, which is a different shade to your facial skin tone. If the foundation blends in completely so it is hardly visible it is the right shade for you.

Foundation is extremely noticeable when applied in the wrong shade or not properly blended. Do avoid the orange line at the edge of the face and do not try to alter your skin colour/tone by using a darker shade which can be very aging and a lighter one that can make you look unwell. Colour can be added later with bronzers and blushers.

Bronze skin tones come in more than 35 variations of colour compared to about 10 for ivory skin so bronze skin tones may need to customize their foundation by mixing two shades together for the best match.

Foundation is designed to provide an even skin tone, cover blemishes and protect the skin not be noticeable for everyone to see. Some foundations have additional benefits such as sun protection (SPF), added vitamins and light reflecting particles.

What Kind of Foundation to Use

Liquid:

Liquid foundation is perfect for most skin types and it will cover evenly and fill dips and folds in skin

Tinted Moisturiser:

A tinted moisturiser combines a little colour with a moisturiser to provide a sheer coverage.

Soufflé,

A Souffle foundation provides heavier coverage but is still very light to feel

Cream

A cream foundation comes in both stick and cake form. It goes on thicker and can provide a sheer finish

Mineral Powder Foundation

Mineral Powder foundation is suitable for all skin types. The zinc oxide ingredient is anti-inflammatory, so it is ideal for rosacea and skin blemishes. There is no talc in these foundations to they help to retain moisture and retain hydration. A little goes a long way.

When applying makeup make sure the skin underneath is dry. Then apply with a large flat brush and use circular movements to place into skin.

Pancake

Pancake foundation is for stage use (It is heavier makeup applied with water and a cosmetic sponge)

Oil Free Foundation

Designed for oily skin

How to Apply Foundation

Foundation can be applied with a cosmetic make up sponge, a foundation brush or with clean fingers. Start from the centre of the face and blend outward and upwards into the hairline and along the jaw line. It's personal preference whether to blend down the neck, all depending on variations in skin tone. The whole face should look even and smooth. Apply with a light touch to avoid rubbing off any concealer you've applied. Less is more. You can always build up coverage by applying a second layer, if needed. You may want to apply foundation to the eyelids to provide a more consistent base tone all over the face.

How to Apply Concealer

Concealer serves 2 functions: either to camouflage or to highlight. It usually comes in small containers and is only used sparingly on the face. Coloured concealer can be used to counterbalance discolouration on fairer skin tones. Red can be neutralized by green, pink by pale yellow and rosy by pale lilac.

To apply dab a small amount on what you're trying to hide and blend in. Be careful to use a colour that is not too light, which will have the opposite effect and draw attention to the area. To hide dark under eye circles choose a concealer that is one shade lighter than your foundation, dab onto the dark circle and blend outwards into the foundation application. Dab foundation over the top of the concealer. Blending is key to successful application.

How to Apply Face Powder

There are two main types of powder:

Fine Powder

The most popular powder is translucent as this sets the foundation but doesn't change the colour

Compressed Powder

Found in a compact, is more dense in colour and used for touching up or as a base colour

Application

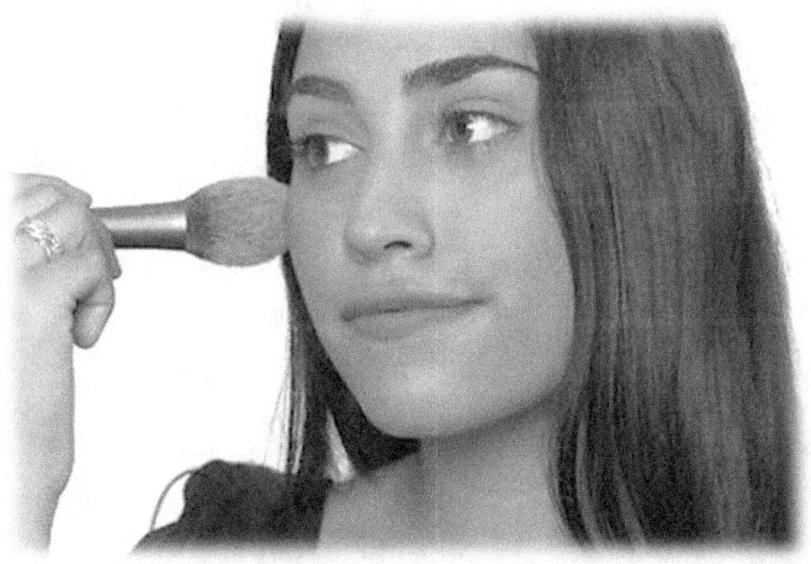

Apply the powder to a clean ball or cotton wool and lightly dust over the face.

Turn the cotton ball inside out and gently brush downwards over the face to flatten the hair on the face

A powder brush (wide fat brush) can be used instead of a cotton ball

When using compressed powders use light movements over the face or the finish will look 'cakey'

Eye Shapes and Makeup Application
Proportioned

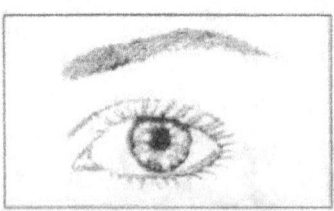
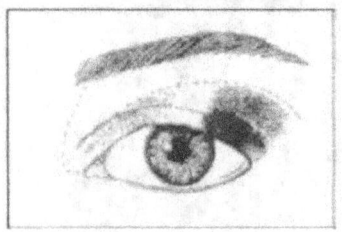
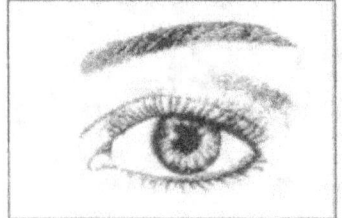

On the proportional eye shape the lid and brow bone are balanced. Usually you have a bit more brow area than lid, but the lid shows. Cover the entire area with highlighter. Then apply a contour shade to the orbital bone, a deeper shade to the outer corner of the lid and a pale shade to the inner lid.

Eyeliner – line the outer half of both the upper and lower lids, feathering a smaller amount of liner towards the nose, to prevent the line ending abruptly. Emphasising the outer half will 'widen' the eyes. Some proportioned eyes have a lot of lid showing as well as lots of brow area. Use a neutral rather than a bright colour on this type of lid.

Little or no lid showing, more brow area

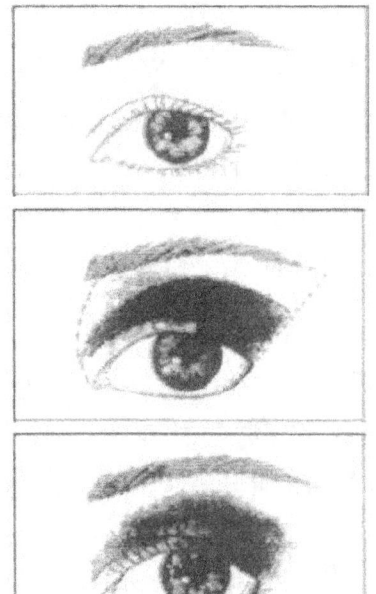

This type of eye has little or no lid showing, with a wider brow area. Asian eyes should consider themselves in this category, as well as hooded eyes or prominent orbital bones.

Apply highlighter to the entire area and then contour shade on the orbital bone, bringing it higher in the centre and extend it a bit closer to the nose, creating almost a semicircular shape. Having shadow higher in the centre will 'open' the eye and prevent a droopy look at the outside edge. Accentuate the outer corner of the eye with a deep shadow and bring out the lid with a touch of pale colour above the iris.

Get Your FREE Gift ...See Page 154

Eyeliner – Line the entire lower lid to emphasise the bottom of the eye but line only the outer third of the upper lid to keep it 'open' and make the eye look bigger.

Little or no lid showing, small brow area

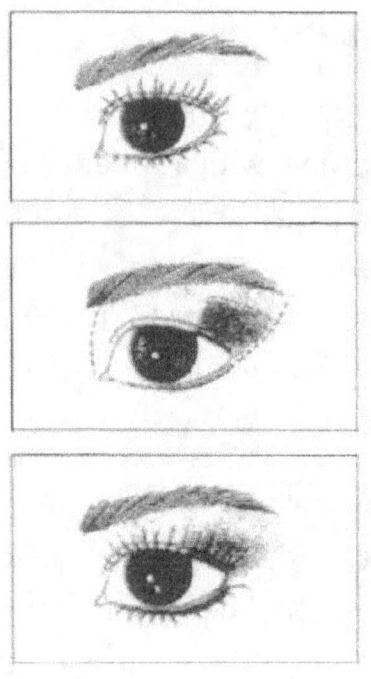

This eye has very little space on which to apply makeup. Apply a pale colour to the entire eye from lashes to brow. Contour the corner with a deeper shade on the outer third of the lid, swept slightly up towards the outer half of the eyebrow. Do not contour the orbital bone. A light up lifter dot can be placed on the centre of the lid right over the pupil close to the lashes to catch the light and make the iris look bigger.

Eyeliner – Line the entire lower lid to emphasise the bottom of the eye. Lining the upper lid will close in the eye.

Prominent lid, small brow area

A lot of lid shows and is often a larger area than the brow bone.

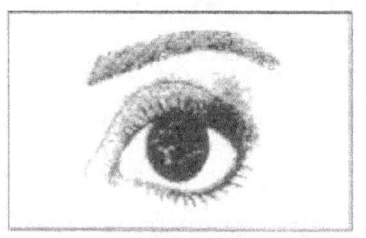
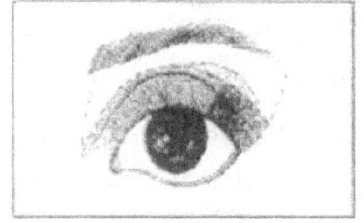
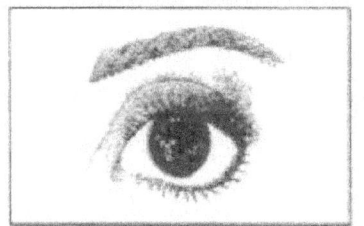

Apply a pale shade across the entire orbital bone blending it towards the eyebrow. Then apply a subtle, medium neutral colour to the inner two thirds of the lid, to recess the lid. If the crease is dark and sunken stop the eye shadow short of the crease. This trick will help make the lid appear smaller and the brow area larger. Now brush a little of a darker shade from the outer corner of the lid up towards the end of the eyebrow feathering it at the outer edge of the orbital bone.

Eyeliner – Line the entire upper lid almost to the tear duct to recess the lid a bit, but line only the outer third or the lower lid feathering the edge so it doesn't end abruptly. Use a medium neutral rather than a dark or bright colour.

Get Your FREE Gift ...See Page 154

Then blend the line to soften it. Be subtle. Everything shows on this type of lid

How to use Eyeliner, Mascara and Eye Pencils

Eyeliner

Eyeliner is available in cake, liquid and pencil form. It is used to define the shape of the eye and give the appearance of opening them up. Depending on the effect desired it is placed on the top, bottom or both lids and either encircles the entire eye or is used on the outer edges only. Softer liners such as cake or pencil can be smudged using a sponge tipped applicator or a cotton bud giving a softer definition to the eye.

Eyebrow Pencils

Eyebrow pencils are used to add definition to the eyebrow area as well as balancing and infilling missing areas of eyebrow. They come in various colours including grey, brown, blonde and black.

To apply brush the brows into shape then use light feather strokes on the brow hair itself to define them. Brush through after application.

Mascara

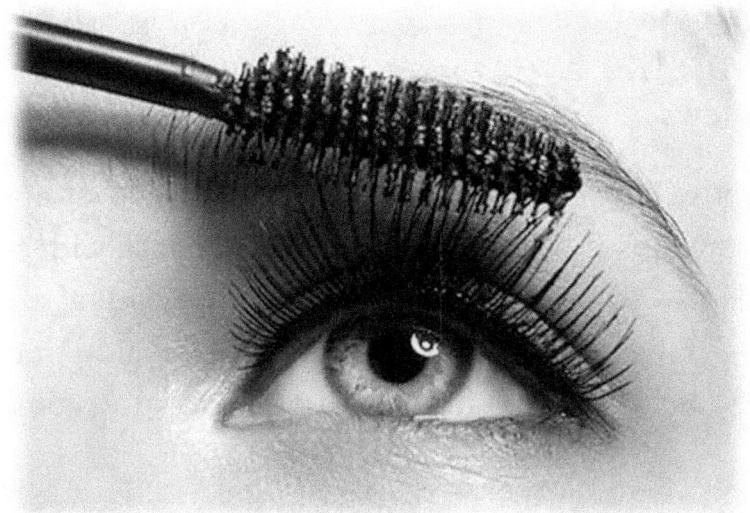

Mascara is used to give definition to the eyes by thickening, lengthening and darkening the lashes. The most popular is the liquid mascara: Black, brown, and a variety of fashion colours.

Formulations

- Waterproof
- Smudge-proof
- Lash lengthening
- Protein enriched
- Thickening

Safety tip: Do not pump the wand in and out of the mascara tube as you are pumping in air which results in it drying out quicker and can introduce bacteria potentially leading to eye infections.

Make up the Eyes
Eye Shadows

The purpose of eye shadow is to accentuate the eyes and make them look brighter – to coordinate the face with an overall look – to complement or contrast the natural eye colour – comes in nearly every colour and finish from matte to shiny. You'll need a range of colours to choose from.

Types

Powder

Powder eye shadow is the most common form of eye shadow and is easy to apply

Cream

Cream eye shadow tends to crease on the eyelid.

Cream to Powder

A combination of the above two which is applied as a cream but dries to a powder.

Wide pencil form

How to Apply Blusher

Blusher adds colour and vitality to the face, giving definition where there was none. Blushers come into many different colours and tones – the most common being pink, peach, purple and brown tones. Most blushers are now in powder form but you can still use cream blushers underneath foundation. Powder blush is more easily blended and can create a more natural look.

Placement

The right placement of blusher is as important as intensity of colour. Apply it too low and the face can look droopy. Apply it too high and too close to the eyes and it can give the impression of being punched in the face.

1. Using either a blusher brush or a clean cotton ball add a little blusher

2. Apply blusher along the cheekbone right under the outer edge of the iris. Place two fingers next to your nose to start and sweep upwards and outwards from there.

3. Blend the colour out the hairline at the tip of the ear.

4. Bring the colour slightly downwards into the hollow of the cheek

5. Blend all the edges so that there is no distinct line where the blusher ends

Using Blusher to change Face Shapes

Narrow

Widen the appearance of the face by starting the blusher at the outer corner of the eye and blending the colour straight back to the hairline at the centre of the ear

Wide

Slim the appearance of the face by blending the blusher slightly more upward towards the hairline just above each ear and a smudge lower than the nose at the other end.

Round

To reduce the roundness of the face avoid accentuating the shape. Do not place blusher on the apples of the cheek, instead softly sculpt the cheekbones in the cheek hollow.

Square

To add more curves apply blusher to the cheek apples in small circular movements

How to Apply Highlighter

Highlighting is a process of using light colours to bring out features and darker colours to minimize them.

Areas that need highlighting include: the bridge of the nose, the cheekbones, and the top of the forehead, the bone under the eyebrow, the eyelids and the tip of the chin.

Contouring or Shading should be applied to the sides of the nose, near the hairline, on the temples, under the cheekbone and in the crease of the eyes.

Foundation is applied everywhere else. All of the areas are then blended together to create a gradual transition from one area to the next.

Lip Products

Lipsticks

Coming in a vast array of pots, wands, sticks and pencils in a wide assortment of colours lipsticks are used to define, enhance and balance lip shape.

A lipstick should be chosen to enhance the makeup and reflect the colour of the clothes that are being worn

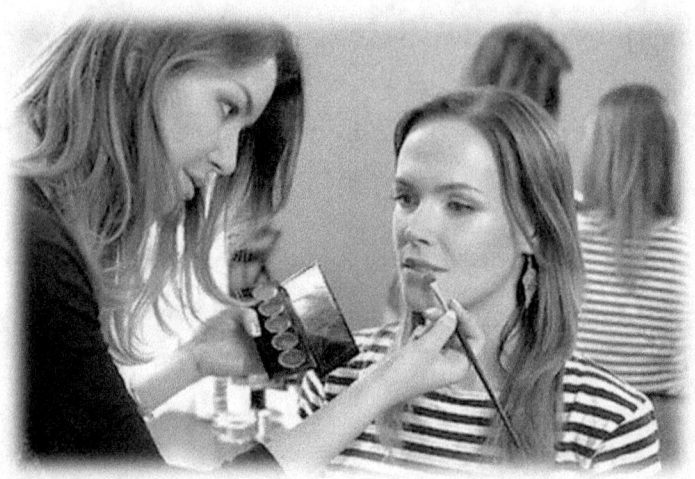

Lip gloss

Gloss can be clear or pigmented and used under or over lipstick or on its own depending on the effect required (semi-shine or full on shine) Glosses are not as durable as lipsticks and need reapplying. They come in wands or pots. Used to add sheen and sparkle to the lips after or instead of the application of lip colour.

Lip Liners and Pencils

These are used to outline the lips. Pencils are good for correcting the lip area by balancing or realigning the lips. They also help in stopping the 'bleeding' effect around the mouth

Finishing the Look

You may want to finish your work by setting the makeup with finishing powder brushed lightly over the whole face. Translucent powder is good for this as it sets the makeup and prevents shine whilst leaving the colour of the makeup unchanged. Avoid placing powder on the eye or lip area as doing so could dull the colours used in the makeup.

Airbrushing

I myself never used airbrushing to do makeup but it can be used to great effect. Makeup, particularly foundation is sprayed onto the client in a fine mist using a small compressor, a hose attachment and a pen-like tool.

It can produce a more natural looking makeup that lets the client's natural skin tone shine through. A look online will provide you with more details about training courses and suppliers.

> *"Makeup is a way for a woman to look and feel like herself, only prettier and more confident"*
>
> *Bobbi Brown*

Customer Care: Consultations, and Keeping Records

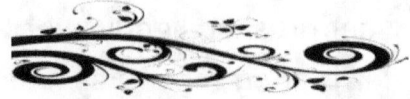

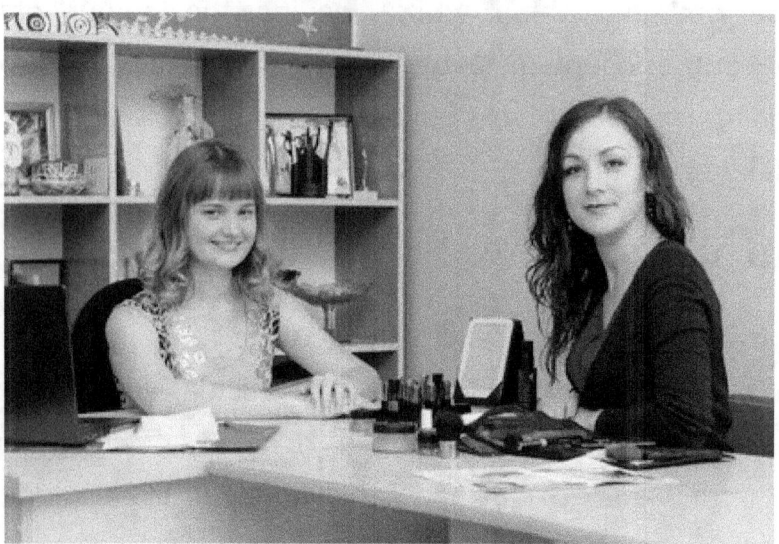

In order to have a thriving Makeup Artistry Business you need to show exceptional customer care. Your client will return to you over and over again and will be happy to provide a testimonial and refer others to your business if what you provide is considered valuable and outstanding.

Everyone wants to feel special and makeup in particular is tied up with your client's self-confidence. By making your customer look fabulous they will feel fabulous and their confidence will soar. A great perk of being a makeup artist I feel is to be able to make your customers feel special.

How to Conduct a Customer Consultation

A customer consultation is a way to establish trust with your client as you discuss with her how she wants to look. The consultation is where you find out more about the client, her lifestyle, her personal style and any event coming up for which she wants to look fabulous. It's a time to discuss skincare, colours, allergies and special requirements and concerns.

It is essential that you carefully listen to what your client is saying. Everyone wants to be heard and you need your customer to know that what she says is important to you. In addition you want them to be relaxed and comfortable which makes the makeup application a lot easier to do.

Welcome your client when they arrive or say hello if you are going to their home or place of work and introduce yourself to them if you haven't met.

Give your client a consultation form to complete as well as a pen whilst you set up your makeup area, tools and supplies.

Answer any question your customer may have

Once the consultation form is complete take a look at it and familiarize yourself with what your client has written.

Ask additional questions if any information provided isn't clear to you. Ask open ended questions about her lifestyle, her personal style and any events coming up.

Ask about her skincare routine, colour preference, any allergies and any special requirements and concerns. Has she had a previous makeover? If so what did she like and not like about it.

Listen carefully to the client's answers and maintain eye contact throughout the consultation. Add any notes you want to add on the consultation form.

Be supportive and respectful, sensitive to your client's privacy and personal details. Be aware of the Data Protection Act.

Design a makeup for your client and discuss what you are going to do.

Do what you said you were going to do and perform 'your magic' transformation being polite and friendly whist you work. Avoid inappropriate conversations.

You can find examples of customer consultation forms on the website at http://makemoneywithmakeup.com

- For a makeup application session.
- For a bridal makeup application session
- For a Special Occasion

In addition to the questionnaires above you'll also need to make some notes about your client's features and other makeup needs to help you in your makeup application.

The Client Assessment Form.

During the Makeup Application Session itself write down notes about what products you use, the colours chosen and placement of the products. This is particularly important if you need to recreate an identical look on a later date.

A face chart is useful to illustrate your notes. This enables you to show exactly where products were placed and the colours and shades used: A useful tool for a client following a makeup application session and also for you when you conduct for example a bridal trial which might be several months before the actual wedding.

One final form that is useful to have pertaining to the makeup session is a client feedback form. These can be used as testimonials to aid in your marketing. Use as quotes on both your brochures, business cards and on your online marketing materials such as your website.

For more information on customer care take a look at the resource section at the back of the book and visit our resource page at makemoneywithmakeup.com

Creating a Unique Identity for your Makeup Artist Business

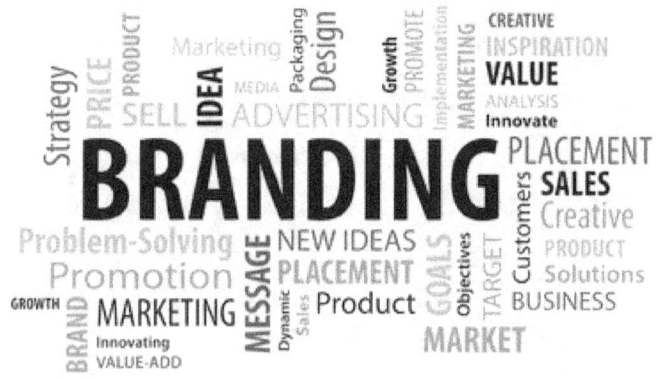

The biggest question on a makeup artist's mind is usually "where do I find customers for my business?" The answer to this is In order to get clients for your business you have to be very clear about what you can offer them and what makes you different from all the other beauty professionals in your town or city. You have to stand out from the crowd. You want to be the first person people think of when they are looking for someone offering your types of services and/ or products in your local area.

One of the ways to stand out is through your unique identity. Your image: In other words your brand. What do potential customers think about when they look at your business? More importantly what would you like them to think about you when they look at your business? Carefully planning and then implementing your brand and using that brand consistently throughout all your marketing materials and within your business dealings will ensure that you are creating a unique identity for your beauty business: A unique identity that sets your business apart from the all the other similar businesses, a unique identity that attracts clients to your makeup artist business.

Your Business Vision and Mission

First and foremost let's take a look at your business vision and mission.

Vision – What's the big picture for you and your business? What do you see in your future? Where do you want your business to be in one year, five years, and ten years? Do you envisage growing your business or staying small? Do you want to hire others to work with you or work alone? Do you want to offer additional services and products in the future? If so what? Your business vision gives you a chance to dream. To really look at what you ideally want your beauty business to look like in the future. Having an idea of where you are heading really helps you put in place the necessary steps to get there.

Mission – The mission for your beauty business explains the purpose and philosophy behind your business. Do you want to specialize in any particular skill area for example wedding makeup or hair? Your purpose and philosophy could be to ensure that each bride you work with enjoys a relaxing experience that provides a time of peace and calm on her busy day. A well-crafted, authentic mission statement provides a strong foundation for your business plans and marketing efforts.

Your Brand Name

To be unique and to stand out from the crowd you and your business need to be memorable. Spend some time choosing a name that is memorable. One that is:

- easy to remember
- easy to spell
- web friendly (important these days)

Check that your proposed business name:

a) Can be registered as a domain name (available website name)

b) is available on social media sites

Tip: Do you want to be known in a specific geographic area? Include that area in your name (this will help in being found more easily online)

Your logo

Your business logo is a visual representation of what your business stands for. Potential customers can instantly know what your business can offer them. A good logo can provide a professional look and feel about your business and help establish your brand identity.

There are three types of logo:

- A font based logo such as IBM (using written letters)
- An illustration based logo such as a makeup brush or hair dryer
- A graphic symbol such as Nike's swoosh

When creating your logo think about how to convey your brand in a way that is simple and easy to understand.

Other considerations for a logo include:

Your message - Is your business fun or more formal for example. Each quality will require a different kind of logo

Differentiation- How can you make your logo stand out from the logos of your competition?

Get Your FREE Gift ...See Page 154

Functional – How will your logo look like at different sizes and on different mediums from the smallest product label to the magnetic strip you might add to your car. What will it look like on your website?

Font style – Is the font suitable for your business name? Is it a flowing design or a more formal one?

Your Brand Promise

What promise are you making to your customers that both really matters to them and makes you different from your competitors? It is essential to attracting new customers and instilling loyalty amongst your current customers that you stick to your promise. Your brand promise is the emotional statement that you make to customers that identifies what they should expect in all their dealings with you. It is often called a 'tag line' and should evoke a positive emotion.

Don't be afraid to make a promise. If you are confident in your skills and your ability to give your customers a memorable experience you will more easily stand out from everyone else and be the beauty business of choice. Your customers want to know that when they come to you they will receive the same excellent service and/or products. They want a consistent experience.

In order to be the beauty business of choice ask yourself what promise your brand makes and what purpose it serves to your customers. Once you've made this promise look at everything you do in your business and make sure that every customer experience is congruent with this promise. If it is your clients will love you and you won't need to be concerned about the competition.

Your Brand Purpose

The importance of building a brand on a purpose, not simply a promise helps consumers understand what the brand stands for: Your reason to be. Your greatest strengths and what you have to offer. It highlights what you provide the market, how your business is different, and what makes your business distinct.

Your Brand Personality

Your brand personality is how you want to be seen by your customers and potential customers. What set of human characteristics most closely represent your customer's experience?

For example do you want to be seen as:

- young, upbeat, spirited, exciting, and imaginative or sincere, honest and genuine

- reliable, responsible, dependable and efficient or
- sophisticated and glamourous?

You can show your brand's personality through the products you use, the services you offer, the uniform you wear and what you specialize in. By adopting a brand personality that most closely resembles your personality you will create a stronger connection with your customers and potential customers. Those who love what you have to offer will choose you above everyone else. Be different. Be unique. Be you and draw customers who want that experience to you.

Your Brand Consistency

When implementing your brand it is critical that you use it consistently. The last thing you want is to create mixed messages to your customers. Brand consistency is achieved when you maintain a uniform image and identity throughout your beauty business and products / services. The consistency helps to keep your brand vivid and recognizable. The result of brand consistency is a cohesive and unified marketing front that gets real results.

Make sure that your brand is demonstrated clearly and consistently in your:

Get Your FREE Gift ...See Page 154

- Social media profiles
- Website
- Blog name
- Email signature
- Phone message
- Networking associations

Your brand is who you are, what you represent, and what makes you and your business unique and different from your competition. Spend time creating your business brand and working through this checklist to ensure a comprehensive and clear brand – a brand your prospects won't be able to resist.

For more information on branding your business take a look at the resource section at the back of the book and visit our resource page at makemoneywithmakeup.com

Attracting Clients to Your Business

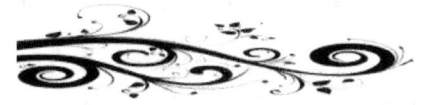

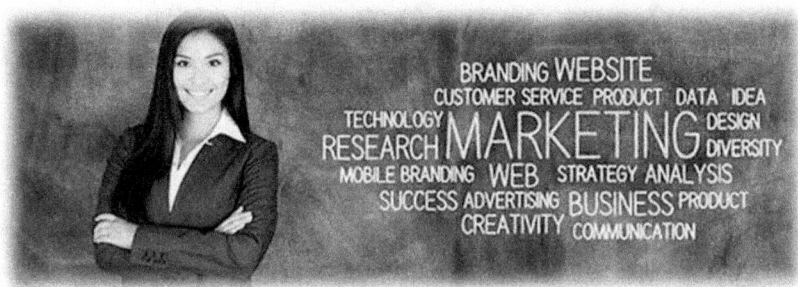

In this chapter we are going to be looking at how to attract customers to your business. You may love your work as a makeup artist but unless you become good at marketing and promoting your skills and your business you won't have enough clients to continue. However you feel about selling learn to be comfortable about it. You have a skill that makes your customers feel special so let the world know about it.

First Steps

Before you decide how you are going to get clients for your business you must understand your 'target market'. Simply this means 'who is more likely to be your customer'. By knowing who is more likely to be your customer you can save both time and money by directing your marketing at the right people. Earlier we looked at the importance of finding the right customers; in other words 'your target market'.

If you haven't done so already write down who is your customer. What type of makeup artistry do you want to do? Who would make your 'ideal client'? When you know who you want as your ideal client think about where you would find them. What do they read? Where do they shop? What websites would they visit? Where do they hang out in social media? Find out as much as possible about them. Once you know where to find your clients you can direct your marketing efforts where they will see it.

There are two main categories of marketing these days: offline and online. Take a look at both of them then decide on which 2 or 3 ideas only that you want to start with and take massive action. Put them into practice as quickly as possible so you can see which of the initial action steps you take works best. If an idea doesn't work for you or doesn't work as well as you expected simply analyse how you could improve upon it or drop it and

Get Your FREE Gift ...See Page 154

select another. Speed is important. Don't keep doing the same thing over and over. If it's not working drop it and try something else!

Offline Marketing

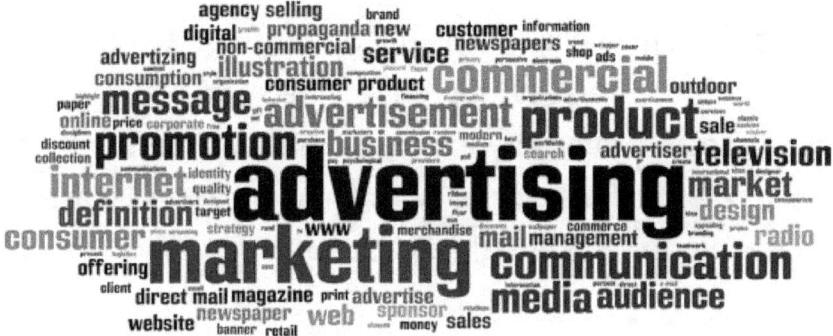

Newspaper Advertising

An expensive form of promoting your business and results can vary but if you've got the budget to advertise in a newspaper consistently it can work. Make sure that the newspapers readers are your target market though. A newspaper ad that isn't seen by potential customers will be no good whatsoever and will be money wasted.

One type of newspaper advert that may work better is one placed in a special 'bridal spread'. At certain times of the year a newspaper may run a two or more page spread or even a pull-out section specifically focused at brides and weddings. This would be a possible time to promote a bridal makeup service.

Magazine Advertising

Similar to newspaper advertising magazine advertising is an expensive form of advertising. However, if you plan to run a premium makeup artistry business and your ideal client reads a certain type of magazine then it might be a good place to promote your business. For example there are a lot of bridal magazines which may be a good place to promote a premium bridal makeup service.

Bridal Fairs

Another way to promote your makeup artistry business to brides and their wedding parties is at bridal fairs. Prices for a stand vary widely and you can have mixed results. If the weather is bad and there are a lot of bridal fairs advertised in your local area then from my experience the results are poor.

However, if you do the research and find a bridal fair that has a good turnout of your potential customers it may be a worthwhile investment. Ask other traders if the bridal fair is helpful to their business. One or two well attended and well known bridal fairs a year, despite the cost of having a stand there, may well provide enough clients for the year. This may be a better investment than attending a lot of lower priced smaller bridal fairs.

When considering the investment required, potentially running into the hundreds, look at the possible return to your business. In other words can you earn enough from each client who meets you at the bridal fair to do the job and make a profit?

Yellow Pages

Have you noticed the size of your 'yellow pages' recently? At one time 'yellow pages' was the place to advertise your products and services. However, with the development of the internet, 'yellow pages' in book form has suffered substantially from a drop in customer advertising. If you can get a very good deal it might be worth considering. However, think about how you search for products and services. Do you use 'yellow pages'?

Local Directories

If your customers are primarily based in your local area then a local directory will give your business exposure. It is said that people have to see your business logo or something to do with your company seven times to make an impression on them! There are so many advertising messages out there today that you have to be seen everywhere to get known.

When advertising in a local directory or even a newspaper of magazine (as outlined above) include a call to action. An ad that doesn't ask readers to do anything will not succeed nearly as well as one that gets the readers to actually take action. Provide a telephone number for people to call in exchange for something of value. It can lead to an answering message set up for the purpose of getting people's details.

Once you have their details you have a list of prospective customers you can call and promote your business to.

Press Releases

Press releases are a great way to promote your business at low or no cost. Send one to local reporters at least once a month to promote your business. Include a great headline which creates curiosity (think about what headlines attract your attention!)

You can send a press release to let people know that you are opening your business, adding a new product or service, attending a certain event, doing some work for a particular charity and other newsworthy events.

Direct Mailings (e.g. leaflet dropping)

Direct Mailings are a great way to promote your business in the local area. Create an ad on A5 paper or use your business card and either deliver them yourself or hire a distribution company to deliver them for you. If you've got teenagers wanting extra money that might work too!

Make sure to add a call to action in the ad or on your business card and use to build your list of potential customers.

Leave brochures and business cards in wedding-oriented businesses like bridal consultants, bridal shops and caterers, hair salons, trendy boutiques and dress shops.

Whenever you publish photos of your clients make sure you have a signed model release form giving you permission to use the images in any of your promotional materials.

Speaking to People

Speak to people everywhere you go. Build up relationships. Strike up a conversation and use FORM (speak about their family, their occupation, and their recreation) this way you'll know whether they fit your profile of an ideal customer! Then give your message: let people know that you are in business and what you have to offer. You can always say "it may not be for you but do you know anyone who may be interested in what I have to offer?"

Networking Events

If you are new to an area then attending networking events may work for you. The purpose of networking events is to get known. Don't use them just to hand out your business cards to everyone there. You come across as pushy and put people off finding out more about you. Again your aim is to build relationships with people. Get to know them and as mentioned earlier use FORM. Getting involved with the events or networking clubs themselves will increase your profile potentially leading to more jobs.

Asking for Referrals

The better you become at providing a wonderful and unique experience for your customers the less you have to 'sell' your services. Your customers will do that for you. A business built and maintained through referral marketing is the ultimate goal. Don't forget to ask for referrals and you could even offer something of value in exchange for names and details of potential customers. Provide an exceptional service and customers are more likely to want to share these with you.

Cross Promotion

Particularly helpful in marketing a bridal makeup artistry business cross promotion involves promoting your services alongside another business. Is there a wedding shop for example that is willing to promote your services in exchange for you promoting them? If offering specialist makeup services for disfigured clients you could cross promote with a plastic surgeon or oncologist. Get to know local event planners and party planners! Contact local vendors who you want to be associated with.

Charity Work

Choose a charity and offer to do free makeup services for them. Perhaps host a pampering evening for them or a fashion show where you apply makeup on the models. You'll get known and your message is likely to be shared by the charity. You can share details of the evening with a press release too. Working with a charity can help to build your reputation in the local area.

Fish bowls

A fishbowl can be very successful if placed somewhere frequented by your ideal customer. It is simply a bowl of box where you can collect business cards or provide a small survey for people to fill in in exchange for something of value; perhaps a drawing for a makeover. You can contact everyone who provides their details whether they won or not to let them know about what products and services you provide.

Give Talks and Demonstrations to Local Women's Groups

Generate interest in your makeup artistry business by giving talks and makeup demonstrations to local women's groups. Leave behind business cards and speak to those attending about what you do and 'who they know' who might be interested in what you do!

Write an article or column for a newspaper, magazine or newsletter.

By writing an article or column for a newspaper, magazine or newsletter or online an article, blog post or guest post you are increasing your reach. In other words the more you put yourself in the public eye the more people will hear of you and potentially the more business you will get.

Teach a Class, do a workshop or hold a Makeup Party

If you're passionate about makeup and love to talk to people about what you do why not teach a class, do a workshop or hold a makeup party. You can earn extra money, show your knowledge and skills and again the more people get to know you the more successful your business will be.

Online Marketing

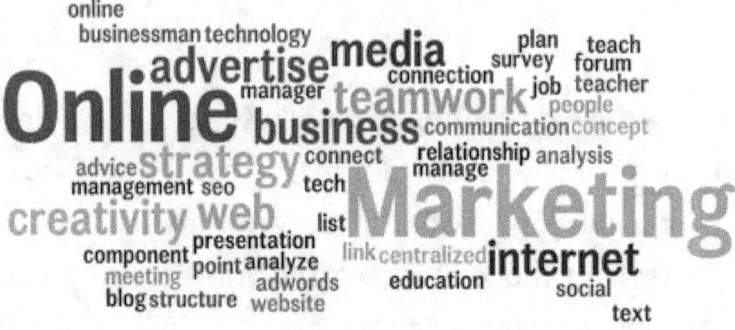

There are all sorts of ways you can advertise on the internet either inexpensively or for free. Once set up you can also leave it to advertise for you.

A website is a must. Your website is your virtual storefront and the best way for people to find you. People are searching for makeup artists on Google. Are they going to find you?

Website

You have 3 seconds to get the attention of your website visitor. Ask yourself what questions you would ask if you were a customer and provide the answers for them.

- What services do you offer?
- How much do you charge?
- How do I contact you?

Website Must Haves:

- A Great Headline
- Pictures and/or Photo Gallery
- Video
- Rates Page
- Contact Page
- FAQ Page
- Testimonials Page
- About Us Page
- Areas you Cover
- What Service you Offer
- Lead Capture Device (a way to get names and email addresses)
- Great Content

Once your website is set up you also need to consider how you are going to promote your website online so it is seen by people searching for your products and services in your local area.

Social Media

Social Media is a great way to showcase your talent as a makeup artist and spread the word about what you do. The aim is to draw people's attention back to your website for more information about what you offer. People love images so why not post photos and create albums of your work, post behind the scenes photos of you working, offer makeup application tips, offer specials and run contests and promotions, and link to other websites where your work may be featured.

Interact and connect with others: wedding planners and photographers, other makeup artists. Show an interest in their work and make comments on their social media sites. Get known. Be friendly.

It is important not to be pushy on social media. You want to be seen as offering valuable information and being helpful. Readers are put off when their social media feeds are full of advertising and they will unfriend you if you come across that way.

If you need greater details about attracting more clients online visit http://makemoneywithmakeup.com for current courses on offer. The main thing about online marketing and promoting your business on the internet is that it is always changing and progressing as technology advances. Standalone marketing courses are designed to keep you up to date with what works today in promoting your beauty business online or offline.

Are **you** ready to start your own makeup artist business? I hope that now you've reached the end of this book that you'll understand that you too can follow your dream, become a makeup artist, set up a home based business and make money with makeup. **You can do it!**

We've looked at some foundational principles and built upon them as we got into the practical aspects of setting up your own makeup artist business. We've looked at the ingredients for success as a makeup artist business owner, the qualifications needed, business planning, legal, insurance, money and tax implications, how to create a winning beauty portfolio, what makeup to choose, tools and supplies to do the job, health and safety, services to offer your clients, customer care, and last but not least how to attract clients to your business..

The next step involves you. I would love to hear how you are doing in setting up your own home based makeup artist business. Do let me know by emailing me at anne@makemoneywithmakeup.com

Get Your FREE Gift …See Page 154

Useful Websites

Makeup Magazines
Makeupmag.com
Cosmeticsbusiness.com
Makeup411.com

Page Makeup Charts
Amazon.com and .co.uk
Thefacechart.com
karla-cosmetics.co.uk/

Makeup Artist Portfolios
Zazzle.com
portfoliomart.com/
cassart.co.uk
portfolio-store.co.uk

Online Beauty Retailers
Cinemasecrets.com
Camerareadycosmetics.com
Getthegloss.com
Myshowcase.com
Beingcontent.com
Lookfantastic.com
Threecustom.com
Victoriahealth.com
Thisisbeautymart.com
Lovelula.com
Cultbeauty.co.uk
Beautybay.com
Allcosmeticswholesale.com
Dextermakeup.com
Bobbibrowncosmetics.com
Benefitcosmetics.com
Maccosmetics.com

Toofaced.com
Thebalm.com
Urbandecay.com
Esteelauder.com
Makeupforever.com
Tartecosmetics.com
Stilacosmetics.com
Gurumakeupemporium.com
Sephora.com
Ulta.com
Bennye.com
Evepearl.com
udshop.com
Viseart.com
Graftobian.com
Kryolan.com
Coverfx.com
Mehron.com
RCMAmakeup.net
Yabycosmetics.om
Alconeco.com
Ballbeauty.com
Lecosmetique.com
Makeupart.net
Preciousaboutmakeup.com
Sigmabeauty.com
Starsmakeuphaven.com
Avon.co.uk
Marykay.co.uk
Mallatts.com
Bhcosmetics.com
Coastalscents.com
Elfcosmetics.com
Jordanacosmetics.com

Milanicosmetics.com
Makeupgeek.com
Nyxcosmetics.com
Rubykissescosmetics.com
Sallybeauty.com
Sleekmakeup.com
Shanycosmetics.com
Thebeautystore.co.uk
Feelunique.com
Xtras.co.uk
Beautyexpert.com
Lookfantastic.com

Community websites
Makeupalley.com
Temptalia.com
Modelmayhem.com
Hmartistnetwork.com

Education
beautyschoolsdirectory.com
makeupgeek.com
youtube.com
makeupmag.com
delamaracademy.co.uk
makeupacademy.co.uk
nasmah.co.uk
habia.org
themakeupchair.ie
themakeoverstudio.com
eproimagecourses.com
qcmakeupacademy.com
robertjonesbeautyacademy

makeuponlinetraining.com
makeupmentors.com
hmartistnetwork.com
airbrushmakeup.com
kettcosmetics.com
temptupro.com
airbasemakeup.com
artistswithin.com
blanchemacdonald.com
cinemamakeup.com
cmucollege.com
ei.edu
joeblasco.com
libsbeautyschool.com
makeupschool.com
mkcbeautyacademy.com
schoolofmakeupart.com
promakeupart.com
studiomakeupacademy.com
skinandmakeupinstitute.com
vfs.com
westmoreacademy.com
debramacki.com
elanmakeup.com
jlsmakeup.com
themakeupshop.com
vanessamills.com
brushstroke.co.uk
iveracademy.co.uk
thelondonmakeupschool.com
beauty-school.co.uk
centralschoolofmakeup.co.uk
londonmakeupacademy.co.uk
theacademyofmakeup.com

glaucarossi.com
bammakeup.com
brightonmakeupschool.co.uk
themakeupschool.co.uk
aofmakeup.com
schoolofmakeup.co.uk
aquarosamakeupschool.co.uk
thesessionschool.com
londonmuse.co.uk
make-up-school.co.uk
cassielomasmakeupacademy.co.uk
makeupschool.com.au
makeupcollege.com.au
cameronjane.com.au
makeupcourse.com.au
makeup-college.com.au

huxleyschoolofmakeup.com
academyofbeauty.com.au
nida.edu.au
makeuptraining.com.au

Tradeshows
Imats.net
Umae.co.uk
Themakeupshow.com

Business Skills
Hmartistsnetwork.com
Makemoneywithmakeup.com

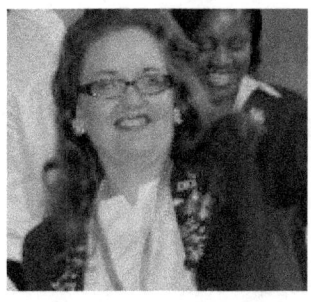

About the Author

Anne Perez, former international makeup artist and team leader with two cosmetic giants. I am currently a writer, speaker, coach, marketer and entrepreneur and am passionate about helping others live life with passion: A life by design rather than default.

I have had the pleasure to have taught and mentored hundreds of entrepreneurs, professionals and business staff in makeup artistry, marketing, IT and entrepreneurial skills.

It's great to be able to manage my own time. Yes I work hard but I also have time to travel, visit with friends and family, follow my hobbies and be generous to others.

However you want to live your life stop dreaming and take action. You can do it! If you want to contact me just drop me a line at anne@anneperez.com

A Closing Note from Anne

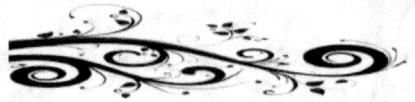

As you can probably tell I love to help business owners set up and grow successful businesses. One of the ways to become successful is with online marketing. If you are interested in discovering how to attract more customers to your business then I have a very special free gift for you.

I want to invite you to a free online and on demand training I have for you called

'How to Attract Customers Today through Online Marketing'

This is a complete step by step training that is in fact FREE and you can even ask questions.

All you have to do is navigate over to
http://www.yourinternetmarketingguide.com.

Check it out now and you could have new customers by the end of today. Really!